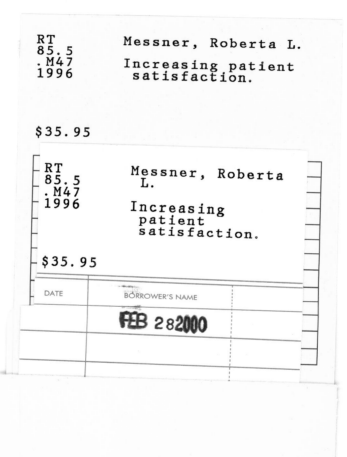

RT
85.5
.M47
1996

Messner, Roberta L.

Increasing patient
satisfaction.

$35.95

RT
85.5
.M47
1996

Messner, Roberta
L.

Increasing
patient
satisfaction.

$35.95

DATE	BORROWER'S NAME	
	FEB 28 2000	

Increasing Patient Satisfaction

Roberta L. Messner, RNC, PhD, CPHQ is certified in medical-surgical nursing by the American Nurse's Association and in healthcare quality by the Healthcare Quality Certification Board. The recipient of many national writing awards, she has published over 700 articles, short stories, books, and chapters in professional and consumer publications. She has participated on a number of advisory boards for nursing/medical journals, and currently serves on the editorial board for *R.N.*

Susan J. Lewis, RN, PhD, CS, is a Psychiatric Clinical Nurse Specialist. Dr. Lewis has taught numerous workshops on the national level and has published extensively in a variety of nursing and medical journals. She and Dr. Messner are co-editors of *Manual of Psychosocial Nursing Interventions,* which was awarded an AJN Book of the Year Award in 1989. She is also coauthor of *Managing the Violent Patient: A Clinician's Guide.*

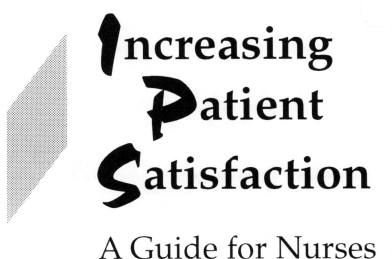

Increasing Patient Satisfaction

A Guide for Nurses

Roberta L. Messner, RNC, PhD, CPHQ

Susan J. Lewis, RN, PhD, CS

SPRINGER PUBLISHING COMPANY

Copyright © 1996 by Springer Publishing Company, Inc.

All rights reserved

No part of this publication may be reproduced, stored in a retrieval system, or transmitted, in any form or by any means, electronic, mechanical, photocopying, recording, or otherwise, without the prior permission of Springer Publishing Company, Inc.

Springer Publishing Company, Inc.
536 Broadway
New York, NY 10012

Cover and interior design by Tom Yabut
Production Editor: Joyce Noulas

Second Printing
97 98 99 / 4 3 2

Library of Congress Cataloging in Publication Data

Messner, Roberta L.
      Increasing patient satisfaction: a guide for nurses / Roberta L. Messner,
Susan J. Lewis.
            p.   cm.
      Includes bibliographical references and index.
      ISBN 0-8261-9250-5
      1. Nursing—Quality control.   2. Patient satisfaction.   3. Nurse and patient.
I. Lewis, Susan (Susan Jane)   II. Title.
      [DNLM: 1. Patient Satisfaction—nurses' instruction.   2. Quality of Health
Care—nurses' instruction.   W 85 M5851 1996]
RT85.5.M47   1996
DNLM/DLC   95-25628
for Library of Congress   CIP

Printed in the United States of America

Contents

*For my dad, Jim Hogsett,
the grandest storyteller of all*

— Roberta

For Cindy, Johnny, and Shangool

— Susan

Foreword

As the editor of a national journal for nurses, I read lots of other newsletters and journals in the healthcare field. Recently, they were full of discussions about healthcare reform, both legislated (which didn't happen) and de facto, resulting when American business turned to managed care in a big way.

Virtually all the discussions centered not only on providing healthcare we as a country could afford, but on assuring that it was quality healthcare. The only problem is, no one is yet able to define quality. For one thing, we need standard outcomes measurements to define clinical levels of quality. There are lots of groups working on those, and the only problem will be figuring out whose parameters are best.

But we also need to define the quality of the nonclinical care patients receive—the caring, if you will. It's nurses who provide much of that caring and, in overseeing nursing assistants, housekeeping, and others influence most of the rest of it. Time after time, patients list nurses right there at the top as determinants of a positive healthcare experience.

If we know who determines the quality of the caring, we don't have a definition of what goes into that caring. Exactly what is it that a nurse does to make the patient feel cared for? In point of fact, we never will have an exact definition, because each patient is an individual, and what pleases one immensely will be ignored entirely by another, and may even irritate a third. But we'd sure better start trying to pin down some basics—some attitudes—that make for patient satisfaction. In a cost-driven environment, when technical quality is a given, it's service that keeps customers coming back.

Roberta Messner and Susan Lewis address the problem in this book, and, indeed, go a long way to solving it. I have never liked the trendy term "client" and have never used it when referring to patients. It seems far too sterile. I think of ad agencies and attorneys who are out only to finagle the most they can out of a deal. Messner and Lewis, however, use the term "customer" to refer to patients, and I don't mind that. It states the essence of patient-centered care, and taking cues from business—as Messner and Lewis do—on how to please the customer makes very good sense in today's healthcare environment.

In some institutions, there will have to be radical attitude adjustments to convince staff that they need to find out what motivates people—read patients and customers—and give it to them. For many nurses, however, the return to an emphasis on caring will be very welcome indeed.

This book serves as an important orientation tool for adjusting attitudes that need adjusting. With any luck, it can help spark enough change so that I won't ever again have to write in an editor's memo that by "forgetting the nursing arts courses learned back in the '30s, too many individuals are leaving patients and their families shaking their heads and yearning for the nurses who used to 'care.'"

— Marianne Dekker Mattera
Editor, *RN*

Acknowledgments

This book was prepared with the help and encouragement of many people. Special thanks is extended to:

Henry Gernhardt, Jr.
Ruth Chasek, Nursing Editor, Springer Publishing Company, patients, families, and healthcare workers who shared their experiences.

Introduction

The average American, during his or her lifetime, will spend 49 hours seeing doctors and 64 hours waiting to be seen (Heymann, 1991). Like many people with a chronic illness, I've far exceeded those figures. The year I turned 15, I was diagnosed with neurofibromatosis, at that time known as "The Elephant Man's Disease." At an age when my peers were consumed with the excitement of boys, fashion magazines, and ball games, I experienced painful and disfiguring tumors, failing vision, seizures, and fainting spells. I might have disappeared into despair had it not been for my remarkable mother who truly believed that opportunity could be found in my adversity.

A serious genetic, neurological disorder? Yes. A catastrophe? No. Mother, a former elementary school teacher, and I traveled from one specialist to another, seeking a diagnosis and care for a problem which had no known cause or cure. While I missed months of school, she made it her mission to transform clinic waiting areas, hospital rooms, and bus and train depots into classrooms. Whether we found ourselves in rural Amish country or a large metropolitan city, we studied the experts around us. I wrote about it all in my diary. "Pay attention to the people," Mother would often say, "there's a lesson here."

If I was talking to a man who had had open heart surgery 5 years before, I would find myself asking: "What do you remember most about being in the hospital?" Or, if I was waiting to have a brain scan, and the lady sitting beside me mentioned she was scheduled to begin chemotherapy, I would wonder out loud: "What helps you get through it?"

It has been 26 years now, and my curiosity about patients' perceptions of healthcare has only grown. Back then, before dreams of becoming a registered nurse held the slightest promise of reality, I recognized that nurses—the frontline caregivers—were the vital coordinating center of this complex thing called healthcare. I also observed that people, as a rule, trust nurses. A patient's interaction with a laboratory technician or even a doctor is generally very time- and procedure-limited. But nurses are with you over the long haul when no one else is around.

I will carry the memory of many of those moments with me forever. When I was a patient on pediatrics at a well-known medical center, my brand new graduate nurse, Patty Oakley (we dubbed her Annie Oakley, after the western heroine) would entertain us by bouncing quarters on freshly made beds to demonstrate the tautness of the linens. "Annie" was new to much of the technology of nursing, but she was a natural when it came to communicating with frightened children and teens. If Annie said we should "ambulate, pardner" or eat all our vegetables (to the musical score of "Annie Get Your Gun," of course), we did it gladly. She made us feel special, and we simply adored her.

Annie "sold" nursing the way McDonald's sells hamburgers. Even with her inexperience, she knew that the secret of caring for patients is *caring* for patients. With consumer confidence in healthcare slipping, it is a message that bears listening to today.

In these 26 years (21 of which have been invested as a nurse in clinical, educational, research, administrative, and editorial roles), I have continued to be a consumer, provider, and student of healthcare. I have noticed that most nurses work extremely hard, but that doesn't necessarily mean we satisfy patients and their families. I have observed as well that it is not enough to give high quality care if patients don't perceive it as excellence provided with a genuine respect and concern for them as persons.

The demands on tomorrow's nurse will be greater still. We must prove our worth by being multiskilled, and even more flexible, and by mastering the difficult art of doing more with fewer resources. And past successes don't promise future ones.

In the not-so-good old days, quality was considered a luxury for some, rather than an expectation for everyone. But today's healthcare customers are much better informed and expect more. And with quality under the microscope, regulatory bodies are insisting that healthcare agencies measure two dimensions of quality: clinical outcomes and customer satisfaction. That's right: patients' perceptions are now considered an important gauge of quality. For it is customers who ultimately decide whether to purchase our product —healthcare—from us again. And while many patients are ill-equipped to accurately judge the quality of their care, they are fully capable of judging the quality of their caring.

Like the nurse who cornered me at a community hospital the other day, you, too, may contend: "When they started calling the patients 'customers,' I didn't like that. This isn't a dime store. A hospital can't run like a corporation." But the future of quality healthcare is largely determined by our business savvy and by viewing our organizations as "an interrelated system rather than a collection of discrete programs and services" (Joint Commission, 1994, p. 1). "Historically," says Sovie (1994, p. 30), "our [health care agencies] have been organized to serve the clinicians and the departments, not the patients and their families."

Maybe this doctor's words will sound familiar: "All this change isn't patient-driven. It's money-driven." Perhaps so. But nurses have been saying for years that healthcare isn't really responsive to patient needs. And we have wanted to delight, not merely satisfy, those we serve. At long last we have a forum. Administrators and providers at all levels are finally giving more than lip service to some of the issues that matter most to us, and to those matters of the heart that never change. The exciting end result is that improving the performance of a healthcare organization is now an interdisciplinary, collaborative process for which all caregivers share accountability.

Admittedly, it was a little disquieting the first time I heard patients referred to as customers. It seemed to somehow diminish the multifaceted roles we nurses juggle. But to be honest, I have come to respect the term. To me, it symbolizes that paying attention to the *customer* is *customizing* their care. I like the sound of that. For those of us who don't focus on our customers will soon be out of business.

The content of this book reflects an extensive review of the professional and lay literature, including lessons gleaned from industry; patient, family, and provider interviews; and my continuing personal journey from both sides of the bed rail. Its nine chapters are written for both practicing nurses and students, and address the major issues that affect patient satisfaction with healthcare.

Today, patients are as much disturbed about poor communication as poor treatment. A strong thread throughout the text is that medical/nursing care is largely interactive; therefore, caregivers must master the art of rapport and sensitive communication.

As you read this book, you will likely find yourself saying "I know that" or "I've been saying that for years." And for good reason, as this book reflects the collected wisdom of many generations of nurses. As you read, take time to reflect on your own stories.

Chapter 1 poses the book's central question: "What Do Patients Really Want? (It May Be Different Than You Think)." Customer expectations represent an increasingly complex phenomenon, with numerous variables influencing what patients expect from their healthcare providers. This chapter explores actual patient examples as well as pertinent research on customer perceptions and their "great expectations."

Chapter 2, "The Changing American Healthcare Scene and Patient Satisfaction," takes a long, hard look at current issues and trends on the healthcare horizon. Clearly, healthcare systems that package their services with their customers in mind will be more successful in the future, and will face less litigation as well.

Chapter 3, "Quality Isn't a Coincidence," examines healthcare in light of a comprehensive, practical approach to continuous quality improvement (CQI). Pertinent Joint Commission on Accreditation of Healthcare Organizations (JCAHO) standards and dimensions of quality are demystified, and strategies for using patient satisfaction data to improve organizational performance are presented. These concepts are woven throughout the book as well to demonstrate how the CQI culture is synonymous with empowering all levels of staff to produce a quality product.

All patients have the right to be treated as unique individuals in an atmosphere of respect, acceptance, and trust. Privacy, confidentiality, and the right to active participation in the decision-making process are among the issues reviewed in Chapter 4, "Yes, Patients Do Have Rights."

While effective patient education facilitates healthy behaviors and timely discharge, thereby saving healthcare dollars, ineffective efforts may result in preventable readmissions and unhealthy behaviors, and increase costs. Chapter 5, "Patient Education: A Key to Increased Satisfaction," will enhance the nurse's ability to comprehensively address patient/family education and discharge planning needs.

Patients all too quickly lose their identity in today's healthcare milieu, and can assess the healthcare environment with amazingly astute perception. Chapter 6, "Creating a Hospitable and Healing Environment," will help nurses establish a warm, therapeutic atmosphere regardless of their practice setting.

While a satisfied customer may express that satisfaction to four to five people, a dissatisfied customer will complain to 20 or more (Press, Ganey, & Malone, 1991). Chapter 7, "How to Handle a Customer Complaint," will demonstrate effective strategies for problem resolution and for transforming a negative experience into a positive one.

Chapter 8, "Measuring and Evaluating Patient Satisfaction Findings: Looking for the Lesson," demonstrates that every complaint presents an excellent learning opportunity, as patient satisfaction data compel us to examine our own behavior and weaknesses. Nurses are in a central role to elicit and evaluate patient feedback. The Appendix features a sample patient satisfaction survey based on the major tenets of this book.

Lastly, Chapter 9, "Be Kind to Yourself and Your Coworkers: A Plan for Enhanced Morale and Patient Satisfaction," turns a much needed corner to ponder the personal and professional needs of today's nurses and their impact on customer satisfaction.

What do patients really want? Ask yourself that question in your daily nursing practice. The answers may sometimes surprise you, but should always guide you.

Someone once challenged Helen Keller to imagine a predicament worse than being blind. Her thought-provoking response? "Having good eyesight and no vision."

No one knows precisely what changes still await us in healthcare. But one thing is certain: customer satisfaction is our vision for the future, and it begins with you.

Mother and Annie Oakley were right.

References

Heymann, T. (1991). *In an average lifetime.* New York: Fawcett Columbine.

Joint Commission. (1994). Important functions debut in mental health manual. *Joint Commission Perspectives, 14*(4), 1.

Press, I., Ganey, R. F., & Malone, M. P. (1991, Feb.). Satisfied patients can spell financial well-being. *Healthcare Financial Management,* 34-42.

Sovie, M. D. (1994). Nurse manager: A key role in clinical outcomes. *Nursing Management, 25*(3), 30-34.

Chapter 1

WHAT DO PATIENTS REALLY WANT? (IT MAY BE DIFFERENT THAN YOU THINK)

Don't be internally focused. Learn what's important
to customers and clients.
— Richard A. Moran

As I shopped for a birthday gift for my little nephew, I found myself drawn to a captivating display of expensive oak and brass kaleidoscopes. The perfect present, I quickly decided; when I was growing up I'd always wanted one myself. I would imagine spending hours designing fascinating colors and shapes, all with just the flick of my wrist.

I couldn't wait to ask my sister how her son was enjoying the gift of my dreams. "I don't want to hurt your feelings," she answered, hesitating, "but he's played more with the box than with the kaleidoscope." While I had the best of birthday intentions, my efforts fell short of success. The reason? I purchased that gift because *I* liked it, and not because it was right for him.

There's a lesson in that little incident for the all-too-common stories we hear these days about patient dissatisfaction with healthcare:

- A first-time mother complains that they sent her home from the hospital before she knew how to care for her newborn. "Nobody even listened when I told them my

1

husband was out of town and our closest neighbor lives
2 miles away," she explains. Four days later, the infant
is readmitted for dehydration.

- A business executive with angina contends he can't find
  a doctor anymore who "really explains things." Weary of
  complicated medical terminology (his degree is in marketing), he pretends to understand everything, then
  thumbs through his trusty home remedies book for
  answers.

- An elderly lady with a new diagnosis of diabetes tells
  how she waited by the telephone all day for a promised
  return call from the outpatient clinic. She loses faith in
  "all those medical people" because of that one frustrating experience, and decides to "play it by ear" in the
  future.

The list goes on and on. With all the technological advances in
healthcare, it's tempting to assume that we know what our
patients—our customers—need. And because we care and want
the very best for them, it's all too easy to superimpose our values
on those we serve.

WHAT IS PATIENT SATISFACTION?

Patient satisfaction is the degree of congruency between a
patient's expectations of ideal care and their perception of actual
care received. Products and services promised by the media are a
barometer by which expectations are gauged.

Healthcare customers expect to receive quality care at the best
monetary value available. They want professional competence, accurate diagnosis, state-of-the-art treatment, and no preventable complications that might result in a longer hospital stay or prolonged
recovery, disability, or death (Consumer's CHECKBOOK, 1992).

Many consumers, however, feel ill-prepared to assess these
highly technical issues. Just as important, but often overlooked,
are those expectations that aren't so easily pinpointed, yet con-

tribute greatly to consumer confidence (Kirk, 1993). By and large, patient satisfaction with healthcare is related to the "ordinary" human virtues of communication, sensitivity, respect, dependability, trust, and personalized service. In their eyes, we should never become so mesmerized by the extraordinary that we bypass the ordinary.

Nurses play a key role in the larger healthcare picture, and make a critical impact at every turn. And because we are the largest and most visible group of healthcare professionals, the public (and even some fellow providers) tend to equate satisfaction with healthcare in general to the care nurses provide.

In one study, 50 patients who had been hospitalized were asked to describe an experience when they felt cared for by a nurse. Eight secrets of satisfaction were identified (Brown, 1986, p. 58):

- Recognition of individual qualities and needs

- Reassuring presence

- Provision of information

- Demonstration of professional knowledge and skill

- Assistance with pain

- Amount of time spent

- Promotion of autonomy

- Surveillance

While patient satisfaction (and dissatisfaction) is a highly complex and individualized variable, patients expect outstanding care from caring people (Scott, 1993). Here are some specific concerns gleaned from the literature and hundreds of our personal interviews with patients and their families (Hsieh & Kagle, 1991; Hill, Bird, Hopkins, Lawton, & Wright, 1992; Gerteis, Edgmen-Levitan, Daley, & Delbanco, 1993; Kirk, 1993; Messner, 1993; Mack, File, Horwitz, & Prince, 1995):

Factors that May Affect Satisfaction with Care

- Customer expectations

- Communication

- Age (elderly patients are more likely to express greater satisfaction with healthcare than their younger counterparts)

- Gender (some studies have indicated that women report greater satisfaction than men, while other studies have contradicted this finding)

- Health status (patients with failing health or chronic illness are often less satisfied)

- Socioeconomic factors (low income decreases access to care and may increase skepticism with the healthcare system)

- Religious beliefs (people with a strong sense of spirituality have greater hope and a belief in the good intent of others)

- Educational level (education empowers people with a greater sense of control and understanding of health and illness)

- Past experiences (of the patient, family, or acquaintances) with healthcare (what other people have told them about a particular disease, practitioner, or institution impacts a person's perceptions, expectations, and response to treatment)

- Continuity of care (fragmentation of care equals dissatisfaction and decreased trust)

- Confidence in the healthcare agency

- Level of current physical or psychological distress (patients in physical or psychological distress have a diminished tolerance for uncertainty and inconvenience)

- Support systems (financial and people)

- Reasonable waiting time

- Accessibility to needed services

- Perceived empathy and compassion of providers

- Coping mechanisms (poor coping skills hinder potential for physical, psychological, and spiritual healing)

- Family-friendly environment

- Current happenings in the patient's personal or family life (additional stressors compound healthcare needs and problems)

- The media (mass media exerts a profound effect on expectations and attitudes)

CLARIFY EXPECTATIONS

To provide customer-focused care, it's crucial to know who your customer is. That sounds simple enough on the surface, but what you must determine is *their* expectations—not merely yours or those of your employer. All too often, we try to sell consumers the healthcare and services *we* want them to have.

It's also important to determine why consumers choose us over our competition. That's a key to understanding what makes your organization unique, and to planning services that maximize customer satisfaction and loyalty. In these competitive times, the goal is to determine your special niche, not to duplicate services already offered elsewhere.

Here's where a comprehensive patient assessment (with input from the entire interdisciplinary team) will help. Simply ask, "What did you come here for today? What are your expectations?

Question further to really understand the patient's needs: "What else did you want to tell me today that I've passed over?" While some will volunteer this information on their own, others may feel intimidated and suffer in silence. Let patients know their input is valued.

"Whenever a new patient is admitted to our unit, I try to assess what they expect as part of my initial nursing assessment," says Mona. "If they're a little shy, to break the ice I often say something like, 'Did you ever get something for Christmas that you couldn't use and didn't even want? Well, we want to serve you in the best possible way. Be sure and tell us what you need.' Otherwise, we spend too much time solving problems patients don't even identify as problems."

Patient-centered care has been defined as "the redesign of patient care so that hospital resources and personnel are organized around patients rather than around various specialized departments" (Staff, 1993, p. 14). How much better than hopping on the latest trend or struggling to provide a program the competing clinic across town is already offering. When you learn what the customer wants, you open the door for merging patients' often surprising expectations with state-of-the-art care—for tying healthcare into what is meaningful for them. Ditto your chances of having a satisfied customer as well as a healthier one.

The elderly lady who hasn't been hospitalized since her last child was born may be thinking nostalgically of the good old days when nurses always offered patients a back rub. If you don't provide that extra touch, she may well perceive you as "that new generation of nurses who have forgotten the basics," even though the actual care you provide may be superb.

No one said it better than Hippocrates in his timeless wisdom: "It's more important to know what sort of patient has a disease than what sort of disease a patient has." There is no high-tech substitute for getting to know our patients and clarifying what they expect from us.

Nursing Sets the Stage

Today's consumers recognize that nurses are pivotal in providing and coordinating healthcare. *Take This Book To The Hospital With You,* published by People's Medical Society, makes this observation: "The person who can help you more than anyone else within the hospital walls, who is there for you more than anyone else, who will look out for you and bend the rules for you, is your nurse" (Inlander & Weiner, 1993, p. 66).

Yet almost never does a patient judge solely the technical aspects of care. Caring, too, is a critical element. Madeleine Leininger (1984, p. 14) said: "Care remains the essence of nursing. . . . Nursing as a discipline will find its place in society and in academic institutions through the explication and use of care." Caring, the "very core of nursing" (Larson, 1984, p. 46), remains a constant in the face of unsettling changes in the healthcare industry.

Still, caring for the patient isn't enough; a patient's family must also perceive us as caring, as Long and Greeneich (1994a) stress in their article about families' perceptions of critical care nursing. They recommend that nurses assess whether the patient's and family's expectations are being addressed in a satisfactory manner.

Although healthcare is routine for us, it is anything but for patients and their loved ones. "Even in the worst of circumstances, it's the nurse who pulls you through," concludes a registered nurse whose daughter recently gave birth to triplets. "The nurses' attitudes established the tone for our whole terrifying experience. When the babies were so fragile during those first few weeks, the nurses told us what to expect, and reassured us that they were making progress. I made up my mind, in the future, I'm going to try to be positive like that. Patients really model a nurse's reaction."

The Impact of the Media

Take a look at *The New York Times Book Review's* best sellers list to see how many book titles deal with the human aspect of modern medicine. Or peruse the pages of popular lay publications many patients read, such as *The New Yorker, Psychology Today, Ladies' Home Journal, McCall's,* and *The National Enquirer.* Titles such as "How To Find A Doctor Who Really Cares" and "Hospitals: Hazardous To Your Health" will tell you what is foremost in the public's mind. In addition, many consumers today own a Physician's Desk Reference (PDR) or medical texts, and will challenge your comments against the volumes on their bookshelf.

By the time a person is 60 years old, he or she will have been subjected to an average of 50,000 ads and 350,000 television commercials (Keen & Valley-Fox, 1989). They are in the habit of changing TV channels on a whim by remote control. Consumers have a low tolerance for unsatisfactory service and inferior quality, and when the hassles overwhelm, many comparison shop as if they were buying an automobile. To be sure, unrealistic expectations are fueled by the media, with today's customer seeking instant and highly personalized solutions, even in healthcare.

In addition, "baby boomers," influenced by the Vietnam War, Watergate, the women's movement, the Cold War, the threat of nuclear annihilation, and the equal rights movement, are vastly different than their depression-era ancestors who value economic security and have a higher regard for authority (Gerteis et al., 1993). In the healthcare milieu, baby boomers want information, choices, and a sense of partnership with their providers. Their parents and grandparents, on the other hand, are more likely to trust and accept healthcare—even the bureaucratic component—without question.

SERVICE: AN OUTMODED IDEA?

The other day I overheard a lady at a pharmacy window complain: "'Customer Service' is just an empty cliché here. They ignore you. This pharmacy might have a good reputation, but they haven't helped me." Yet posted in a prominent spot was a shimmering brass plaque that read: "A customer is the most important visitor on our premises. He is not dependent on us—we are dependent on him. He is not an outsider in our business—he is a part of it. We are not doing him a favor by serving him—he is doing us a favor by giving us the opportunity to do so."

"It's like the furniture store," the lady continued. "I had the cash in hand to buy a chair, and the salesman was amazed when I inquired if the floor model sofa that was falling apart could be repaired. He made no effort to accommodate me, but there was that blasted slogan, 'A Satisfied Customer,' on his desk."

"They shuffle patients around at my doctor's office like shoppers traveling from store to store," complains a patient recently diagnosed with lung cancer. "When you're sick, you don't feel like walking across the street for a blood test, much less down the block for an MRI."

It's no secret that consumer confidence in general is slipping. Cynicism abounds. But when it comes to health matters, it's especially disquieting. The road to customer satisfaction may be paved with good intentions, but if those intentions don't address the specific needs of your customers, they're to little avail. The secret of success in the face of change is found in the word service. Our customers want—and need—to know we're truly at their service.

LISTEN UP

People will tell you what's important to them if you really listen. Be attuned to what's unsaid, too. "I finally found me a doctor who listens," says a convenience store clerk with benign prostatic hypertrophy. "He hasn't done a thing for me yet but pay attention to me and try to understand what I'm talking about. He just holds my hand a little longer, so to speak. I have all the confidence in the world in him because of that. My last doctor would just scribble something in my chart and never even look at me. He was in and out of his office like a whip."

One way we demonstrate genuine concern and respect is by listening. We usually learn a lot, as well. Sometimes we're deceived into thinking that listening takes too much valuable time. After all, in these lean days, every minute counts. But in the long run, taking time to really connect with a patient saves time, and builds rapport (Messner, 1993). If you are pushed, just say, "Mr. Johnson, I only have 10 minutes to talk with you about your insulin today. But I've alerted the other staff that for those 10 minutes I belong only to you."

Listening also leads to improved clinical outcomes. "When our daughter Amy was 4 she broke her leg," remembers her mother, a healthcare administrator. "Unknown to us, within 36 hours she'd developed a pressure ulcer on her heel secondary to the cast. But she was unable to verbalize what was wrong. It was only by listening closely to her cries and watching her move the ice bag from the break to an 'uninjured' heel that provided the vital clues. When the cast was cut off to examine her leg, Amy immediately ceased to cry, with a sigh of relief. On her heel was a deep ulcer the size of a quarter which took 3 months to heal. The doctor said to the nurse, 'Whenever a child cries in pain, listen.'"

Treat each customer like they're your only customer. "Listen with your heart," advises Wilferd Peterson (1993, p. 76). "Practice empathy when you listen; put yourself in the other person's place and try to hear his problems in your heart." Doing so creates a favorable first and lasting impression.

Interestingly, researchers who studied medical interviews found that 69% of patients were interrupted by their physicians within the first 18 seconds of relating their symptoms. Even worse, the majority of interruptions were with closed questions which didn't encourage further discussion. Doctors should be talking less and listening more, the researchers concluded (Staff, 1994).

"I tried to tell my doctor I'd been using 120 supersize pads during every menstrual period for over a year," says a stay-at-home mother with two small children. "My hemoglobin was 6.8, but he just pushed me to the side and said, 'Keep charting your periods so I can see how you're doing.'"

Often we as nurses fall into a similar trap when we try to gather information to complete a form. A far better approach is to ask patients to tell us their story and let the data we need naturally flow. Do not just listen to words, but to the feelings behind those words. You'll arrive at a more accurate assessment of needs and a more on-target plan of care. After all, only 7% of communication is verbal. Thirty-eight percent involves tone of voice, while another 55% is revealed through body language (Willingham, 1992). Really listen. Sure, it takes a little more time, but it's time well invested in terms of rapport, and it communicates a genuine sense of caring. Few people listen well. Those who do really stand out in customers' minds.

What Is the Customer's Superior Need?

Author John Lytle is president of a marketing consulting firm who noticed that managers often spent precious time trying to make decisions based on superficial customer needs. A better question, he proposes, is to ask: What is the customer's superior need(s)? (Lytle, 1993). People often miscommunicate their heartfelt needs due to fear, embarrassment, shyness, or the inability to express them accurately.

To complicate matters, caregivers often misinterpret what their customers are trying to communicate. "If you want to find out what your customers really want, you have to discover what they really need," says Lytle (1993, p. 1). And if you identify and meet the customer's superior need—the one that supersedes all others—you've passed the most difficult test of customer satisfaction. As Ron Willingham (1992, p. 97) explains: "In almost every business or profession there's something you can do that leaves people with an unexpected feeling of joy. The secret is to do something *unexpected.*"

A geriatrics nurse employed in a nursing home remembers: "I cared for a clinically depressed and withdrawn stroke patient who absolutely adored ice figure skating. When we bought her a TV Guide and scheduled her care around the Winter Olympics, she became a totally different person . . . more interested in life and willing to participate in her rehabilitation . . . to do everything she could to get better." You see, the innovative nursing staff tapped into a superior need, and in the process nursing was elevated to an art as well as a science.

We can't assume that just because a nursing intervention is well intentioned, the customer perceives it as caring (Brown, 1986). "We have high standards, we satisfy the criteria of outside accreditation agencies," you might reason, "Isn't that enough?" But to your customers, doing all the "right" things really isn't enough. And working hard isn't necessarily synonymous with satisfying customers either (Scott, 1991).

Patients do experience surprises with their healthcare, and these surprises—good and bad—are important determinants of overall patient satisfaction. In one study, 39% of hospitalized patients revealed they were surprised by some aspect of their experience. The most common bad surprises (a greater predictor of dissatisfaction) were outcome of hospital stay, obstetrics, and baby care, while the most common good surprises were overall quality of care and attitude, attention, and concern from nurses (Nelson & Larson, 1993).

To survive and prosper in today's and tomorrow's changing and competitive world of healthcare requires a different vision. Meeting the customer's superior need results in not merely a satisfied customer, but a delighted one, one who will recommend your services to friends and family, and increase nursing's overall job satisfaction in the process.

MAKE YOUR CUSTOMERS FEEL IMPORTANT

Mary Kay Ash, the founder of Mary Kay Cosmetics Company, attributes her unprecedented success to the ageless golden rule: "Do unto others as you would have them do unto you." A believer that every person is special in his or her own right, she says: "Whenever I meet someone, I try to imagine him wearing an invisible sign that says: 'MAKE ME FEEL IMPORTANT!'" (Ash, 1984, p. 15). It not only helps the recipients feel good about themselves, she observes, but also creates a positive feeling for the person extending that recognition.

In healthcare, the term "customer" isn't limited to patients and families, but encompasses other staff and departments. It's important to accord people inside our organization the same degree of respect and consideration as those on the outside (Scott, 1991).

In past days, it was considered sufficient for those in business to respond quickly and efficiently to complaints about a product. But that is no longer the case. One business study identified that 70% of the reasons why customers took their business elsewhere had nothing to do with product dissatisfaction, but rather with service (Whiteley, 1991). Likewise, customers find fault with our product—healthcare—far less than with the intangibles of their healthcare experience. One way to achieve a competitive edge is to make our customers feel important. Indeed, a lot of healthcare delivery is in the packaging.

"The nurse at our HMO does a fantastic job of anticipating patient and family needs," says Jess, a highly satisfied patient. "It reminds me of how some department stores set up special return counters the day after Christmas. She knows we're going to have questions during off hours, so she started a 24-hour 'Ask a Nurse' hotline. And she set up a system to keep patients posted on things like when they should come in for their flu shots. They're so organized and on top of things over there."

In the hospital setting, scheduling patient care around the patients' familiar routines, and not merely the nursing staff's convenience, is one way to facilitate a caring environment. Ask the patient, "What is a typical day for you?" recommends a case manager on a medical-surgical unit.

"When my mother was dying of cancer," remembers her daughter, a nurse, "the thing that upset me the most was that the hospital staff never reacted to her as the person she had once been. It really taught me to ask patients, 'What was important to you before you became ill? What did you like to do?' It changed nursing for me."

The Ritz-Carlton hotel chain has a unique way of making its customers feel important. Their employees are trained to study customer likes and dislikes, which are then entered into a computer. Upon return visits, personal preferences are distributed to the staff providing services. With this approach, workers at the lowest possible level truly have a voice in customer satisfaction. This idea is not tinseled artificiality. If staff members identify an area of dissatisfaction, they have the authority to correct the problem and spend up to $2,000 on the spot to make the customer happy. As a result, 97% of their customers report having a "memorable experience" at the Ritz-Carlton (George & Weimerskirch, 1994).

Compare that philosophy to the typical healthcare scene, where a half dozen signatures are often required to implement a simple change. Don't forget: patients' expectations parallel what they have come to expect in the business world.

THE IMPORTANCE OF KEEPING YOUR WORD

"If you promise you're going to call me on Tuesday afternoon with my test results, then do it," emphasizes a patient with vaginal bleeding who waited 3 fearful weeks to learn the outcome of her Pap smear. "The receptionist brushed the whole thing off saying, 'I try to follow through, but there's only one of me, you know.' I'll tell you, I'll never go through that cattle run again."

In a study involving over 7,000 outpatients, poor telephone access was ranked as the leading cause of dissatisfaction. This complaint surprised investigators, who found the problem existed in all practice settings they studied (Berwick, Blanton, & Roessner, 1990). Often it's the clerical staff who are responsible for communicating test results or getting back to patients to schedule a follow-up appointment. These individuals need proper education in the importance of keeping their word, and should be competent enough to accurately field customer questions as well. Often the failure to do so falls back on the nurse in the organization.

Have you ever hired someone to do repair work on your home, only to discover that they show up when the mood hits, never calling to explain why they didn't keep an appointment? It doesn't matter how good their work is, confidence is compromised. The best ability, someone wise once said, is dependability. If you fail to get back to patients within a reasonable period of time, you break the bond of trust and communicate the message that they really are powerless in the intimidating world of healthcare (Tanenbaum & Berman, 1993).

Even something as seemingly small as promising a bedridden patient a bottle of lotion or a tube of toothpaste can set the stage for future trust. "If you say you're going to do something, deliver on that promise, even if it means jotting a reminder to yourself," recommends a nursing assistant. One day when I made rounds with him on his unit, a total care patient requested some orange juice and a family member asked for a pillow. "Let me write myself a note so I'll be sure to remember," he said. I could see the relief on their faces when he pulled out his scratch pad.

"I'll call you right back" . . . "I'll be back in a minute." Make sure your word is as good as gold, and your department is a place where promises are kept.

TIPS FROM THE BUSINESS WORLD

While concerns requiring clinical judgment should, of course, always be referred to medical or nursing personnel, the world of healthcare is taking cues from well-run business enterprises. Disney theme parks are a valid case in point. New employees spend four days in intensive training so that everyone from the maintenance staff to ticket collectors can answer customer questions with accuracy right on the spot, and provide excellent follow-up to customer concerns (Baum, 1992).

Look around your facility at the signs posted to guide patients. "A patient was standing right under a sign that said 'Radiology' and staring into space," recalls an X-ray technician. "'Where does a person get an X-ray around here?' she asked." If you see a patient or visitor who has lost their way, take a second to point them in the right direction. How many times in your clinical setting has a patient or family asked you a question you couldn't answer? How did you handle this? If consumers receive extraordinary consideration at an amusement park, shouldn't they expect at least the same from us? Keep in mind, in any setting, proper prior planning prevents poor performance.

Don't Keep Customers Waiting

Ever shop somewhere where personnel acted like they could care less if they had your business? Patients often feel that way, too.

In today's fast-paced world, patients consider time one of their greatest resources. "We're all equal when it comes to our time," says Mark, a real estate agent. "Twenty-four hours for everyone!" Yet the medical profession has erroneously long considered their time more valuable than their customers'. Today, excessive waiting is perhaps the greatest source of irritation for patients (Hill et al., 1992; Scott, 1993).

"The staff at my neurologist's office tell all their patients they have 1:00 P.M. appointments," says an insurance executive. "Then it's like Baskin-Robbins. You take a number. They're very capable people, but when I have to wait 2 hours for a 10-minute visit, I get as mad as a hornet. The whole bottleneck waiting room is filled with angry patients." That setting might have worked for June and Ward Cleaver in the fifties, but this is the nineties. "When you can get your oil changed in 15 minutes, why does it take 2 hours to see a doctor?" asks a patient. "My time is just as important as theirs is."

Neil Baum, M.D., a urologist and expert on medical marketing issues, has developed a system of "informed scheduling." His staff have been taught how long to allow for various treatments and procedures, which has resulted in patients being seen within 20 minutes of their scheduled appointment. If that standard isn't met, the patient receives his services at no charge (Tucker, 1991).

Another annoyance is the prolonged length of waiting time from referral to scheduling of an appointment. One study related this occurrence to patients not keeping their appointments (Mason, 1992). Similarly, in another study, the long wait between admission and the procedure was the most common negative comment expressed by patients who underwent same day surgery (O'Connor, 1991). And any delay that is likely to increase hospital stay (such as surgery being cancelled because a patient wasn't medically cleared) or increase costs, is disquieting—especially among patients who are personally paying for some or all of their health-care expenses.

Is your facility organized around customer needs? One clue to the answer lies in the area of scheduling and patient waiting times. Think about it. "The true test of whether you (and your company) are customer-driven is how you set priorities. If the question, 'How will this affect customers?' is always the first one asked, the chances are good the organization is customer-driven" (Moran, 1993, tip no. 84). Cut through the red tape, the depersonalization, and the automation of healthcare at every possible turn.

INDIVIDUALIZE YOUR CARE

Patients tend to agree that the best nurses are the ones who view the patient as an individual and as a whole person, with a body, mind, and spirit (Britton, 1985). Customers are dissatisfied with "one size fits all" healthcare that really doesn't fit anyone's needs.

Patients and their families long to feel like they really matter, and can sense when we're indifferent to their individuality. "The nursing supervisor flipped off my TV during the extra innings of the World Series because it was '15 minutes after TV hours . . . hospital policy,'" remembers a patient who was admitted for meningitis some years ago, and was paying out of pocket for a private room. "The volume was real low and it wasn't disturbing anybody. Every time I drive past there, I wonder if that woman's ever had to be cooped up in a tiny room for 2 solid weeks." Contrast his experience with that of a pediatrics unit where I was once a patient. One evening, a wonderful nurse arranged a slumber party complete with movies and favorite foods. For one teen who died several weeks later from a brain tumor, it was her *first and last* slumber party.

The literature is full of examples showing that patients have very different needs and expectations. Haven't we all heard unsettling tales of nurses getting so carried away with forms that they ask a male patient the date of his last menstrual period, or an 80-year-old female patient if she'd like a family planning brochure?

DON'T PLAY THE BLAME GAME

How often have you caught yourself saying, "That wasn't my fault. The day shift [or another staff member] should have taken care of it"? An important step toward meeting customer needs is to "own" the problem, even if you didn't create it (Long & Greeneich, 1994b). That's why there are different tours of duty in hospitals. Admittedly, there are employees who consistently "dump" their workload on other staff. But this should be dealt with on an individual level, away from the hearing distance of patients and visitors.

Being part of a customer-driven organization means you take responsibility for problems that affect customers, even if it isn't your fault (Long & Greeneich, 1994b). Resist the urge to pass the buck. If the nurse in your home health agency, whose day off is Monday, leaves a problem for the staff to face first thing Monday morning, it accomplishes nothing but poor public relations to blame that nurse in front of the patient. Take a moment to step back and recognize that problem—regardless of how inconvenient—for the moment belongs to you.

KEEP YOUR CUSTOMERS INFORMED

Customer satisfaction with healthcare is largely related to patients receiving understandable information, and to their feeling of being understood by caregivers (Smith & Sanderson, 1992). Providing education which satisfies our customers not only increases the likelihood that they'll adopt our recommendations, but also that they'll return to our institution for their future health-care needs.

Patient needs vary greatly according to individual situations; elderly and chronically ill patients, for instance, identify patient education and discharge planning as particular concerns. These efforts often determine whether they can care for themselves at home or will require institutionalized or other supportive care (Simpson, 1985).

"Patients are often more worried about the unknown than they are that a procedure is going to be uncomfortable," says a nurse at a metropolitan surgi-center. "They tolerate discomfort so much better if they know what to expect and are approached with honesty."

"Whenever I ask a question about my medicine," recalls an elderly outpatient with debilitating arthritis, "they talk to me like I'm a child. I want to say, 'Do you know what it's like to be an old man? Do you ever stop to think you're going to be old some day?' But I don't. I just complain to the fellows down at the hardware store."

An insightful clerk who conducts presurgical interviews certainly has the right approach. "You can't go fast and have satisfied customers," she says. "Good customer relations take time. Some people have just received bad news about a serious illness and need information presented slowly. In those times, something that was only a misunderstanding can incorrectly get labeled as a problem. If you whisk patients through, someone else will likely have to take more time later on."

RESIST THE URGE TO PATRONIZE PATIENTS

In describing her own experience as an oncology patient, Janet Britton (1985) found that certain types of nurses were more therapeutic than others. The well-meaning "parent" nurse who tells patients that "we" need to eat in order to get better or who refers to patients as "Honey" or "Dear," does little to help them feel in control. Patients want us to talk with them, but they really resent being talked down to (Bader, 1988).

"When I went to have my hearing tested," remembers a piano tuner who suffered hearing loss after receiving long-term antibiotic therapy, "the doctor and nurse were whispering something I couldn't understand to each other. I asked if anything was wrong, and the nurse just patted my shoulder and laughed, 'Now, now, that's just doctor talk.' I didn't like that. I never went back, but I've told a lot of my clients about it."

That establishment just got themselves the most effective type of advertising around—word of mouth. Every time we provide patient care, we're giving a commercial. Moreover, that gentleman will not likely forget the inconsideration and indifference he experienced, particularly when it concerned a healthcare problem that affects his very livelihood. Unfortunately, such negative experiences color every future healthcare encounter.

Do You Really Know Your Customer?

One of the most overlooked aspects of customer satisfaction is staying close to customers to determine what they need and want (Spitzer, 1988). The business world has much to teach us in this realm. Consider this statement in a Lands' End, Inc. catalog (1994): "Giving customers what they want, really paying attention and responding, is the reason Lands' End has been so successful and much imitated over the years." This leader in mail order has made it its maxim to offer customers a level of quality that exceeds their expectations.

Do we, as nurses, do the same? Do we really know our patients, not just who they are today, but who they used to be (Farrell, 1991)? "When my mom was being seen by her doctor for the first time," remembers her daughter, "the medical resident asked her to remove her clothes and put on an examining gown. Mom, trying to worm her way out of a turtleneck shirt, began to chant softly, 'I think I can . . . I think I can.' The resident called me outside the room and asked, 'How long has your mother's mental status been impaired?' I broke out in laughter as I explained. 'She taught first grade for 40 years and relates everything to children's stories. She was just quoting a line from *The Little Engine That Could.*'"

The next time you obtain a patient history, take an extra moment to really get close to the person. Ask them what your department (or staff) can best do to help them. What are their expectations for this clinic visit or hospitalization? What previous experiences (bad and good) have they had with the healthcare system? These will influence their current expectations. A successful car salesman says he always probes to learn about customers' nightmare experiences buying cars. "If you can understand those fears up front, you're way ahead of the game," he says.

It stands to reason that if you know what people expect, you are better able to adjust those expectations to reality and increase the likelihood of satisfaction. The actual experience of healthcare is only one determining factor in whether patients are satisfied. Stay attuned to other individual factors to ward off the danger of assigning patients to stereotypes (Farrell, 1991; Hsieh & Kagle, 1991).

After making rounds on her unit to ask patients what the staff were doing right, a nurse commented: "Patient priorities can be a lot different from nurses' priorities" (Strasen, 1987, p. 89). Patients' satisfaction with nursing care is a factor in their satisfaction with their overall experience, and therefore gives your agency a financially competitive advantage (Lucas, Morris, & Alexander, 1988).

Traditionally, healthcare providers have planned services around what they determined to be important. Today's consumers have great expectations and they expect to have a say in their healthcare. They are better informed, more skeptical (Bader, 1988). We must stay close to our customers to hear that sometimes still, small voice.

OUTCOMES MANAGEMENT

Managing and measuring outcomes is the bottom line in the move toward continuously improving the quality of healthcare. Yet we're only beginning to define what's important to our customers and to balance this customer-centered approach with the desired clinical and fiscal outcomes of providers and administrators. In their informative book *Through The Patient's Eyes* (Gerteis et al., 1993), the authors stress that identifying outcomes pertinent to patients may likely transform our entire way of administrating and providing healthcare. Quality, they say, will no longer be quantified only by strict, biophysical parameters such as how a body system responds to treatment. Rather, it will also be assessed by how individuals perceive the process and product of healthcare in improving their overall quality of life.

The potential impact on outcomes should be carefully examined whenever any organizational change is considered. When St. Joseph's Hospital in Houston, Texas, contemplated integrating nurse extenders into their critical care setting, for instance, they scrutinized the effect that single change would have on quality of care, efficiency, and cost. The result was the development of criteria to demonstrate clinical outcomes and patient, family, and staff satisfaction (Fritz & Cheeseman, 1994).

There are five traditional D's of outcome measurement: death, disease, disability, discomfort, and dissatisfaction (Sovie, 1994). But measuring outcomes in a meaningful manner is rarely easy. For example, outcomes measurement is essential to adequately assess pain control—an important clinical and patient rights issue. Yet such studies are notoriously difficult to design and interpret. At the annual conference of the American Academy of Pain Medicine, experts concluded that while accountability in this practice area is crucial, it is difficult—if not impossible—to apply one set of outcome criteria to all patients experiencing pain. Two alternatives are to calculate an intake score to demonstrate quality of medication received, and to have patients themselves assess effectiveness (Boschert, 1995).

Validating patient/family perceptions and individual experience are at the very heart of evaluating satisfaction with care, as well as decreasing feelings of powerlessness and vulnerability (McLean, 1995). The formerly regarded "intangibles" of quality, such as empathy, compassion, listening, and an environment that fosters confidence and trust, are rapidly moving into the scientific realm. While outcomes research is, at present, in its infancy, and has suffered from insufficient study (Sovie, 1994), it will strongly guide healthcare decision-making in the future. With the burgeoning emphasis on cost containment and maximum utilization of resources, nurses will be challenged to redesign and implement care delivery systems that increase productivity and are economically effective and measurable in terms of clinical and perceptual outcomes (Mark & Burleson, 1995).

Clearly, patients who actively participate in their treatment feel more in control and enjoy more positive outcomes than those who approach healthcare from a passive stance. For instance, surgical patients who receive effective patient/family education and psychological preparation are known to have shorter lengths of hospital stay (by an average of 2 days), decreased pain, and a less eventful post-discharge course, and report greater satisfaction with care (Goldberg, 1995).

While even patients with a similar diagnosis may, of course, be vastly different, and therefore not always comparable in terms of outcomes, the impact of effective communication, emotional support, and dissemination of information can't be denied. Non-compliance with treatment, an outcome issue with myriad potential causes and effects, often suggests a communication gap in the educational process. "I was released from the hospital with three new heart medications," recalls a district sales manager for a clothing corporation. "I listened closely to everything they told me and my wife took notes. But a week later, I wound up in the ER with nausea and vomiting. Only then did I learn that the new medications weren't supposed to be added to the old. That little fiasco cost me a bundle of money and 3 days of lost time from work, including a presentation I was scheduled to give at our national sales convention."

According to Bruce H. Medd, MD (1994, p. 45), ". . . barriers to communication can arise that, if unrecognized, can severely limit the therapeutic potential of the medical encounter." Now more than ever, patient satisfaction and positive clinical outcomes hinge on the effective collaboration of the entire interdisciplinary team, rather than nursing practiced in a vacuum.

References

Ash, M. K. (1984). *Mary Kay on people management.* New York: Warner Books, Inc.

Bader, M. M. (1988). Nursing care behaviors that predict patient satisfaction. *Journal of Quality Assurance, 2*(3), 11-17.

Baum, N. (1992, Feb. 17). Doctors can learn much from Disney about patient visits. *American Medical News,* 32.

Berwick, D. M., Blanton, G. A., & Roessner, J. (1990). *Curing healthcare: New strategies for quality improvement.* San Francisco: Jossey-Bass, Inc.

Boschert, S. (1995). Outcomes studies are difficult, but necessary, in pain management. *Internal Medicine News, 28*(8), 25.

Britton, J. (1985, Spring). Good nurses, bad nurses. *Journal of Christian Nursing,* 12-15.

Brown, L. (1986). The experience of care: Patient perspectives. *Topics in Clinical Nursing, 8*(2), 56-62.

Consumers' CHECKBOOK. (1992). *Consumers' guide to hospitals.* Washington, DC: Author.

Farrell, G. A. (1991). How accurately do nurses perceive patients' needs? A comparison of general and psychiatric settings. *Journal of Advanced Nursing, 16,* 1062-1070.

Fritz, D. J., & Cheeseman, S. (1994). Blueprint for integrating nurse extenders in critical care. *Nursing Economics, 12*(6), 326-331.

George, S., & Weimerskirch, A. (1994). *Total quality management: Strategies and techniques proven at today's most successful companies.* New York: John Wiley and Sons, Inc.

Gerteis, M., Edgmen-Levitan, S., Daley, J., & Delbanco, T. L. (Eds.). (1993). *Through the patient's eyes: Understanding and promoting patient-centered care.* San Francisco: Jossey-Bass Inc.

Goldberg, M. C. (1995). If we're lucky, the patient will complain. *American Journal of Medicine, 95*(2), 52-53.

Hill, J., Bird, H. A., Hopkins, R., Lawton, C., & Wright, V. (1992). Survey of satisfaction with care in a rheumatology outpatient clinic. *Annals of the Rheumatic Diseases, 51,* 195-197.

Hsieh, M., & Kagle, J. D. (1991). Understanding patient satisfaction and dissatisfaction with healthcare. *Health and Social Work, 16*(4), 281-290.

Inlander, C. B., & Weiner, E. (1993). *Take this book to the hospital with you.* New Jersey: Wings Books.

Keen, S., & Valley-Fox, A. (1989). *Your mythic journey.* New York: The Putnam Publishing Company.

Kirk, K. (1993). Chronically ill patients' perceptions of nursing care. *Rehabilitation Nursing, 18*(2), 99-104.

Lands' End, Inc. (1994, November 30). Catalog advertisement.

Larson, P. (1984). Important nurse caring behaviors perceived by patients with cancer. *Oncology Nursing Forum, 11*(6), 46-50.

Leininger, M. M. (1984). *Care: The essence of nursing and health.* Thorofare, NJ: SLACK, Inc.

Long, C. O., & Greeneich, D. S. (1994a). Family satisfaction techniques: Meeting family expectations. *Dimensions in Critical Care Nursing, 13,* 104-111.

Long, C. O., & Greeneich, D. S. (1994b). Four strategies for keeping patients satisfied. *American Journal of Nursing, 94*(6), 26-27.

Lucas, M. D., Morris, C. M., & Alexander, J. W. (1988). Exercise of self-care agency and patient satisfaction with nursing care. *Nursing Administration Quarterly, 12*(3), 23-30.

Lytle, J. F. (1993). *What do your customers really want?* Chicago, IL: Probus Publishing Co.

Mack, J. L., File, K. M., Horwitz, J. E., & Prince, R. A. (1995). The effect of urgency on patient satisfaction and future emergency department choice. *Health Care Management Review, 20*(2), 7-15.

Mark, B. A., & Burleson, D. L. (1995). Measurement of patient outcomes: Data availability and consistency across hospitals. *Journal of Nursing Administration, 25*(4), 52-59.

Mason, C. (1992). Non-attendance at out-patient clinics: A case study. *Journal of Advanced Nursing, 17,* 554-560.

McLean, A. (1995). Empowerment and the psychiatric consumer/ex-patient movement in the United States: Contradictions, crisis, and change. *Social Science and Medicine, 40*(8), 1053-1071.

Medd, B. H. (1994). Barriers to patient communication. *Postgraduate Medicine, 96*(2), 45.

Megivern, K., Halm, M., & Jones, G. (1992). Measuring patient satisfaction as an outcome of nursing care. *Journal of Nursing Care Quarterly, 6*(4), 9-24.

Messner, R. L. (1993). What patients really want from their nurses. *American Journal of Nursing, 93*(8), 38-41.

Moran, R. A. (1993). *Never confuse a memo with reality (and other business lessons too simple not to know).* New York: Harper Collins Publishers.

Nelson, E. C., & Larson, C. (1993). Patients' good and bad surprises: How do they relate to overall satisfaction? *QRB, 19*(3), 89-94.

O'Connor, S. J. (1991). Patient satisfaction with day surgery. *Aust. Clin. Rev., 11,* 143-149.

Peterson, W. (1993). *The art of living.* New York: Galahad Books.

Scott, D. (1991). *Customer satisfaction: The other half of your job.* Menlo Park, CA: Crisp Publications, Inc.

Scott, L. (1993). *It's a dog's world.* Carlsbad, CA: CRM Films Leaders Guide.

Simpson, K. (1985, July/Aug.). Opinion surveys reveal patients' perceptions of care. *Dimensions,* 30-31.

Smith, J., & Sanderson, C. (1992). What makes outpatient attendance worthwhile for patients? *Quality Assurance in Healthcare, 4*(2), 125-132.

Sovie, M. D. (1994). Nurse manager: A key role in clinical outcomes. *Nursing Management, 25*(3), 30-34.

Spitzer, R. B. (1988). Meeting customer expectations. *Nursing Administration Quarterly, 12*(3), 31-39.

Staff. (1993, February 5). Putting patients first. *Hospitals,* 14-26.

Staff. (1994). Doctors should talk less, listen more. *Physician, 6*(3), 3.

Strasen, L. (1987, July). Keeping your patients happy. *Nursing '87,* 89-90.

Tanenbaum, R., & Berman, M. (1993, July). Why even patients who like you will sue you for malpractice. *Physician's Management,* 85-97.

Tucker, R. B. (1991). *Managing the future.* New York: G.P. Putnam's Sons.

Whiteley, R. C. (1991). *The customer driven company: Moving from talk to action.* Reading, MA: Addison-Wesley Publishing Co.

Willingham, R. (1992). *Hey I'm the customer.* Englewood Cliffs, NJ: Prentice Hall.

Chapter 2

THE CHANGING AMERICAN HEALTHCARE SCENE AND PATIENT SATISFACTION

W hen the topic of conversation turns to change, immediately 100 different reasons can be offered as to why nothing needs to be different. The following letter, read at commencement exercises by Keynote Speaker A. Michael Perry (Huntington High School Honors Assembly, May 7, 1991, Huntington, WV) and reported to be from the archives of history, is a case in point:

Dear President Jackson:

The canal system of this country is being threatened by the spread of a new form of transportation known as railroad. The Federal Government must preserve the canals for the following reasons:

1. If canal boats are supplanted by railroads, serious unemployment will result, captains, cooks, drivers, repairmen, lock tenders will be without means of livelihood, not to mention the numerous farmers that are now employed in growing hay for the horses;

2. Boat builders will suffer and toll line, whip and harness makers will be left destitute;

3. Canal boats are absolutely essential to the defense of the United States.

In the event of the expected trouble with England, the Erie Canal would be the only means by which we could move supplies vital to waging modern war. As you may well know, Mr. President, railroad carriages are pulled at the enormous speed of 15 miles per hour by engines which in addition to endangering life and limb of passengers roar and snort their way throughout the countryside setting fire to crops, scaring livestock, and frightening women and children.

The almighty certainly never intended for people to move at such breakneck speeds.

Signed:
Martin Van Buren
Governor of New York
April 1829

This letter from New York State Governor Van Buren, who later became President of the United States, makes it clear that the desire to preserve the status quo and fear of change are certainly nothing new. With so much changing at once in today's world of healthcare, consumers and providers alike are caught in the throws of uncertainty and confusion.

THE CRISIS IN HEALTHCARE: A MAJOR CONCERN

A 1993 survey revealed that 40% of Americans viewed the crisis surrounding healthcare as the biggest problem facing our nation today, even more problematic than education and crime (Clements, 1993). Our personal interviews with hundreds of patients and their families indicate that healthcare remains a major cause of concern.

Here are some of their questions and anxieties:

* "Is someone going to do something to curtail healthcare costs?"

* "All of these changes. . . . How are they going to affect me . . . my children . . . my grandchildren?"

* "Has everyone forgotten about the patient?"

- "In just a few short years, there's going to be a lot more of us older folks. What then?"

- "They shuffle you from one specialist to another. No one really sees the whole picture."

Nurses, too, have their own brand of concerns:

- "Everyone is scrambling for their jobs. It creates an atmosphere of discouragement and mistrust."

- "I spent my career-building years with this hospital corporation. Now they're talking mergers and layoffs. Everyone is so competitive. There's no real job security."

- "The bottom line with all of this is money. All we hear is, 'Don't go over the budget.' They're going to hire more agency nurses. They don't have to pay them any benefits."

- "We don't help our colleagues across town anymore. We used to share our policies, procedures and resources so we wouldn't have to reinvent the wheel. Now it's, 'Don't help those people. They're our competition. We have to stay afloat ourselves.'"

- "They send nurses home every time the census gets low. Five years ago, they recruited me with a $2,000.00 bonus. These days, I don't know how much money to plan on from paycheck to paycheck."

- "Why don't they involve clinical people when they make all these high-falutin' decisions? We know what's practical, what will work for our patients. And what's best for the patient is usually the best economic value, too."

- "How can we ever satisfy our patients with all this emphasis on cutting costs?"

THE CHALLENGE OF CHANGE

There's no question that the American healthcare system is changing fast and furiously, and that money is a primary motivating factor. That former management models have not worked well is evidenced by skyrocketing costs as well as poor access to treatment for large groups of people. In 1986, the Robert Wood Johnson Foundation reported that up to 38.8 million people who needed healthcare during the previous year had difficulty obtaining it (Schiff, Goldberg, & Ansell, 1992). The current preoccupation with the spiraling cost of healthcare follows 4 decades of emphasis on technical quality, availability, and range of services rather than fiscal accountability.

The Chinese have a helpful way of approaching monumental change. For them, the word "crisis" has a twofold meaning: danger and opportunity. They've learned the value of making change their friend, not their enemy. But change becomes especially sensitive and political in the healthcare arena because it represents a rejection of the revered traditions of the past. Yet while there's comfort in the old ways, we can't turn back the clock, nor would we really want to. As Sam Walton of the highly successful Wal-Mart chain once said: "Never get so set in your ways that you can't change."

Admittedly, all change is difficult, even if it's perceived as positive. Change, however, doesn't have to be traumatic at all turns. While the healthcare system is changing at a staggering rate, the basic sound concepts of caring, compassion, competence, and customer satisfaction will assume even greater significance, especially for nurses. And the more poised for change that nurses are, the more we will embrace the opportunities that such changes bring.

The emerging focus on healthcare economics has resulted in a number of cost-containment strategies in the corporate policies and business practices of both healthcare organizations and third-party payers. The Diagnosis Related Groups (DRGs) reimbursement system currently in place in hospitals categorizes patients according to their anticipated consumption of healthcare resources. Patients with similar diagnoses, surgical procedures, age, and discharge status are assigned a particular DRG category as a predictor of costs and length of hospital stay.

"For the first time in this century, healthcare providers and health insurers are subject to intense, rigorous and persistent scrutinizing about the quality and value of what we do," says Lansky (1995, p. 32). Healthcare providers at all levels are at long last understanding their accountability for providing cost-effective care without sacrificing quality and customer satisfaction.

MANAGED CARE

While there is much speculation about the future of healthcare, and while those who follow and forecast trends fail to agree on many issues, most predict that managed care will play a major role. The concept of managed care describes a network in which physicians, hospitals, and insurers strive to control healthcare expenses by "managing" access to medical services (Gatty, 1993). Two types of models fall under this category: health maintenance organizations (HMOs) and insurance plans that cover health services provided by a limited number of hospitals and doctors. Lower charges are offered in exchange for a higher volume of patients. This system is popular with insurers and is viewed by employers and the government as an effective way to reduce annual increases in healthcare expenditures.

Although the processes and delivery of healthcare are under a watchful eye, experts disagree on the precise direction of the winds of change. "Billion-dollar delivery systems operating integrated care programs on a 'for profit' basis will prevail," predicts Johnson (1995, p. 45). Conversely, Brown expects the establishment of massive integrated systems on a non-profit basis that focus on prevention and wellness programs. At the other end of the spectrum, Weil speculates that control of healthcare will be limited to a few powerful systems which will abuse that power, thus causing "a public-utility-type control mechanism" (Johnson, 1995, p. 45).

How Will Managed Care Affect the Consumer?

In a managed care system, there exists the danger that traditional priorities of patient-focused care and satisfaction will become secondary, replaced by cost as the paramount concern. "I fear that such programs will view patients as commodities to be controlled rather than people with highly individualized needs," expresses a nurse practitioner.

A fundamental strategy in the managed care model is to limit patient choices for physician and hospital care in order to control expenditures. As a result, such programs can easily become overly complex, bureaucratic, and impersonal (Johnson, 1995).

Still, Americans believe medical care is a basic right, viewing it as a confidential, private matter that involves personal decisions made in collaboration with their physicians of choice. A recent Gallup poll discovered that "85% of Americans believe that freedom to choose their physicians is the most important element to preserve when reforming healthcare" (Whyte & Beall, 1995, p. 1238a). Most assert that healthcare should not be controlled by distant, impersonal third parties more concerned with costs than care.

The bombardment of the American consumer culture, which began to take hold after World War II, has created a customer who quickly becomes bored, dissatisfied, and cynical. Public opinion—what consumers ultimately expect from healthcare, how many restrictions they will accept, and how much they are willing to spend for this system—will ultimately determine the fate of managed care strategies.

CRITICAL PATHWAYS

The use of critical pathways is another new strategy on the changing healthcare scene (Doyle, 1995). Using an interdisciplinary approach, critical pathways provide a recipe for recommended treatment, including diagnostic tests and medications for selected conditions such as chronic obstructive pulmonary disease, major depression, or myocardial infarction.

"I worry that some health problems will be overlooked because doctors will be discouraged from ordering any additional assessments based on gut feelings or their professional experience," says Maria, a coronary care nurse. Some authorities also express concern that proceduralizing healthcare limits a doctor's freedom in diagnosis and treatment (Berwick, Godfrey, & Roessner, 1990), and that the perceived loss of autonomy may trigger resistance among healthcare professionals. For this reason it is recommended that physicians be involved in developing protocols and standards of care from the outset.

CASE MANAGEMENT

The case management framework was developed to approach both cost and quality through an interdisciplinary design with unit-based accountability of patient and clinical outcomes. This type of program often features a Managed Care Council to facilitate communication of ideas between departments and to decrease territoriality. The Council evaluates established standards of practice and treatment. Coordinated with the use of case managers who are responsible for case-type specific outcomes, this team approach uses a planned care map consisting of the traditional Kardex, a plan of care, and ongoing documentation, with the goal of achieving established standards for quality and cost-containment (Flynn & Kilgallen, 1993). Planned-care maps provide direction for where a patient is expected to be on any particular treatment day, and any deviation in the map is addressed.

Case management appears to be one way of using resources more wisely to promote a higher quality of care by all disciplines. With patients followed across departmental lines, continuity of care, patient education, and discharge planning are enhanced and expedited.

PRIMARY CARE

Primary care is described by the American Nurses Association and the National League for Nursing as advanced practice "predicated on the construct of Primary Health Care, with concepts of direct contact, comprehensive care, case management, prevention, health, and wellness" (Barnes et al., 1995, p. 9). Developed in 1965, primary care offers delivery of a complex set of services which includes both initial contact with the health care system and maintenance care. Nurse practitioners as physician extenders are increasingly providing direct, individualized patient and family care, and also filling indirect roles of patient educator, manager, supervisor, consultant, and researcher, initiating any appropriate referrals.

PRIMARY HEALTH CARE

An assessment of health indices by the World Health Organization and the United Nations International Children's Emergency Fund revealed a need to incorporate economic and social development with health issues. Responsibility for healthcare was reassigned from the traditional focus of physician, as a healer, to a primary healthcare worker, as a partner.

The Primary Health Care Model (not to be confused with primary care) addresses social, political, and economic needs as indicators for the health of populations, as well as individuals. Areas under the umbrella of Primary Health Care include: education, availability of the food supply, basic nutrition, safe drinking water, sanitation, maternal/child health, immunizations, prevention and control of locally endemic diseases, appropriate treatment of common illnesses and injuries, facilitation of mental health, and provision of essential medications (Barnes et al, 1995).

Under this community-based system, nurses are emerging as leaders and managers rather than merely assistants to physicians, a role that   includes supervising non-professional community healthcare workers. This model, which recognizes that health is a fundamental human right, is currently more prevalent in developing countries and in underserved populations in the United States.

COMMUNITY-BASED CARE

The hub of healthcare is shifting from the hospital to the community setting. At the present time, 98% of all medical encounters in the United States take place outside the hospital. The American Hospital Association estimates that in 1995, 75% of all surgical procedures performed in this country will be on an outpatient basis (Shortell, 1995).

As hospital days decrease, more and more healthcare is delivered in an agency or the home. Driving this trend is the fact that home health costs approximately 75% less than comparable care provided in the hospital (RN News Watch, 1994a). Home health visits, in fact, more than doubled from 1988 to 1991. Explains Jane Zanca (1995, p. 1): "Once a final stop, home care is now a way station on a continuum of care with patients moving in both directions—back to the hospital or forward to resumption of work and normal activities, with follow-up care provided in the physician's office—as needed."

"The best place to learn about individuals is in their home environment," says Anne, a home health nurse. "Personal strengths are much more evident. Just look at how much stronger an animal is in their own environment."

Yet with the necessity of both men and women working in today's society, managing a family member in the home presents a challenge. Agencies in the community must be available to provide needed support and services. A valuable lesson can be learned from looking at mental health reform in the 1960s and 1970s. Changes in mental health concepts advocated release of patients from institutional to community living. Very few communities had developed programs and resources to meet the special needs of this population. As a result, there are currently many chronically mentally ill persons living on the streets with no place to go and very few long-term care facilities, group homes, or other supervised living situations available.

ONE APPROACH TO COMMUNITY CARE

In New York City, a community-based program called "cluster care" is used to provide higher quality care through a team approach. Also called a "shared aide model," cluster care is a task-oriented method in which social services direct authorized para-professionals to provide unskilled functions for clients who live in close proximity to each other. This takes one of two forms: in the first, a worker provides services to a client several times in 1 day; in the second, several different workers provide services to one client at different times during the same day, accomplishing one or more tasks. These may include laundry, grocery shopping, and help with activities of daily living (Gray & Bailey, 1995).

IMPLICATIONS FOR NURSING

"Just what do these changes entail for nurses?" you might ask. While fewer nurses will be employed by hospitals, it is predicted that approximately two thirds of nurses laid off by hospitals will find jobs in the home healthcare industry. Nurses with specialty experience will be in particular demand (Zanca, 1995). Those in all outpatient and home health roles will be expected to have a more in-depth understanding of acute care, and be able to apply those principles with great adaptability and critical thinking. They will also require exceptional physical assessment, problem solving, communication, and negotiation skills.

Patients cared for in the hospital will be more critically ill. Nurses in all settings must be more flexible and wear an increasing number of hats, and effectively market themselves to survive and thrive. Approximately 500 BSN nursing programs are launching a managed care curriculum to prepare future nurses. Utilization review, quality improvement, and case management are among the topics included (RN News Watch, 1994b).

For the first time in years, job security in the nursing field has been threatened, as demands on nurses' time escalate. RNs and LPNs are being laid off or having their hours decreased. Benefits are being cut. Nurses are being floated to unfamiliar units more often.

One new buzzword is "cross-training," which means delegating a greater variety of tasks and responsibilities to nursing staff. Duties include performing EKGs, drawing blood for lab values, administering respiratory treatments, and even cleaning beds and emptying trash.

A nurse with 35 years of experience points out: "It seems as if we have taken a giant step backward. When I graduated from school, nurses did everything. We gave meds, did treatments, prepared patient snacks, tidied up the units, and mopped floors. Later the use of ancillary personnel allowed us to spend more time at the bedside. Now it's back to washing beds and mopping."

Fifty percent of nurses surveyed by Meissner and Carey (1994) reported that their hospitals have increased the use of unlicensed assistive personnel. Because more of healthcare will likely be delivered by less-trained staff, registered nurses will assume even greater accountability and liability. This demands that we scrutinize processes for delivering quality and legally sound nursing care, even asking ourselves and each other if there is a better, more efficient way something can be done.

One nurse from a large Indiana hospital reported to researchers that licensed staff were being laid off only to be replaced by high school graduates called "team care specialists." These unlicensed assistive personnel were given a 4-day course on I.V.s, assessment, medications, and vital signs, then "turned loose on the floors" (Meissner & Carey, 1994, p. 36).

A return to the generalist in both nursing and medicine is also a wave of the future. Just as people have come to expect one-stop shopping at their favorite mall, they are attracted to the convenience and practicality of one-stop medical care. A dramatic change from "organ" medicine to "person" medicine is already under way, and nurse practitioners are playing a major part in this redesign. Healthcare of the future will be organized with desired outcomes in clear view, not around departmental turfs, egos, or tradition.

"We want to cling to what is sure," says one unit manager, "but the fact remains, nothing in healthcare today is certain. The challenge will be not change for the sake of change, but change which makes a true difference." But we can't change everything at once. That would be as destined for failure as embarking upon a new fitness program and trying to run 4 miles the first day. With the shifting healthcare paradigm, we must preserve the roles that belong to nursing, yet not place ourselves in precarious situations or allow ourselves to become fragmented.

Basic nursing philosophy has held that the patient is the heart and soul of everything we do. "Most of us chose the profession of nursing because we wanted to provide direct patient care," says a med-surg staff nurse. "But as our numbers decrease and our duties increase, we have less time to spend at the bedside. Our challenge will be to make the time we do have with our patients count."

Kupecz (1994) asserts that in the future nurses will assume the major responsibility for determining a patient's care. But the patient—our customer—is an integral part of that team. It's as Bernie Siegel, M.D. (1986, p. 29) commented about the changes he decided to make in his medical practice: "I broadened my role from that of a mere mechanic to include some of the functions of a preacher, teacher, and healer," he said. "I accepted patients as individuals with choices and options. We became a team."

Nurses will continue to be responsible for assessing body, mind, and spirit, and for making appropriate referrals when treatment of problems in these realms is beyond their scope of practice. They will also provide episodic care in the community setting with nurse practitioners providing chronic health maintenance and other services for health promotion, early detection and treatment of illness, and disease prevention. Bill Moyers (1993, p. 55) makes this observation on the critical need for preventive healthcare: "We don't look at the entire spectrum of healthcare approaches, including prevention and rehabilitation. We say, 'We can cure you,' and we give you something to make you better—but then we throw you back out in the environment, which we don't understand very well, and you get sick all over again. The incentives for a health model rather than a medical model just aren't there."

It is estimated that 60–80% of primary and preventive care traditionally done by physicians can be accomplished for less money by nurse practitioners (Kupecz, 1994). "But so many preventive measures still aren't covered by third-party payers," observes a family practice physician. "Yet the wonderments of technology, they're covered. It just doesn't make any sense. How long would your car or household run without any preventive maintenance?"

COMPETITION

Already we are beginning to see more intense competition for patients, services, and financial resources (Kupecz, 1994). Between 1980 and 1993, 949 American hospitals closed, and admissions decreased 11% from 38 million to approximately 33.5 million (Shortell, 1995). While healthcare costs now appear to be a primary focus, this may likely evolve from a purely financial basis to a combination of cost, quality of service, and quality of care, with quality central to the survival of many healthcare organizations (Berwick et al., 1990) and a more humanized approach to patient care (Johnson, 1995).

Understanding how a patient's subjective experiences affect satisfaction and future intentions to seek return patronage from a particular provider is essential to providing quality care in a competitive environment. Mack and colleagues (1995, p. 7) observe that patients judge a caregiver not only on how well the "transaction is executed, but on how well they are treated." The perception of "caringness" helps decrease anxiety as well as a need to assign blame even for "unavoidable imperfect outcomes" (Mack, 1995, p. 14). Nelson et al. (1992) found that dimensions of patient satisfaction accounted for almost one third of variation in a hospital's profit margins.

FOR SALE: HEALTHCARE

Take a look at the advertisements that fill your mailbox to the brim, the billboards in your town, newspaper headlines, and television commercials. There's no debate, healthcare is a prime-time issue. And patients are no longer recipients of care, but rather consumers of care (Warner, 1992). We now have a questioning consumer, one who is increasingly well informed, who has more choices and "shops" for healthcare, and who feels an increasing sense of entitlement (Press, Ganey, & Malone, 1991).

But there's a critical difference between selling and purchasing the most popular brand of tennis shoes and healthcare: Customers see an ad endorsed perhaps by a celebrity they admire. All of their friends are wearing them, so they buy a pair, too. For the most part, they have their minds made up on the brand and style before they hit the shopping trail. But in healthcare, a customer may seek your services for an EKG, but that individual is much different. That individual won't leave with your service neatly packaged in a box, like the last 500 pairs of tennis shoes a store sold. And healthcare doesn't come with a written warranty.

CUSTOMER-CENTERED HEALTHCARE

A strong customer focus in healthcare represents a dramatic shift in culture and thinking. In the old days, explains Sherman (1993), the patient was viewed as an intrusion. Today, we are beginning to ask the customer how we should be doing business.

Now it's the customer who is right—he or she is king or queen. No longer are the physician's word, policies and procedures considered the ultimate authorities. What does the customer want and need? And how can we deliver those expectations with seamless continuity of care and service, building quality into every encounter?

Remembers one patient who underwent surgery to remove a tumor in his colon, "When my doctor said I could go back to work in 4 weeks, I asked, 'Are you sure?' My belly was killing me, and I do a lot of lifting in my job. He gave me that look that told me: you don't question surgeons. All I really wanted was a little reassurance. I'd never had surgery before."

Jill, whose thyroid cancer is considered cured, relates a contrasting incident: "My doctor is just great. He always spends time talking to me before he even opens my chart. It doesn't matter what's going on outside the room, his attention is totally devoted to me. The last time I saw him, he discharged me from his care. But he asked me to drop him a note each year on my birthday to let him know how I'm doing. Can you imagine that?"

Not unlike the business philosophy of Southern States, which has served customers well since 1923: "Everyone who deals with us should leave each encounter feeling warmly greeted and fairly treated by an honest, professional, well-run business enterprise."

If we only knew how much our life experiences resembled one another's. Fear, worry, love, pain—they're all part of the human condition. As Albert Schweitzer said: "Medicine is not only a science, but also the art of letting our own individuality interact with the individuality of the patient." "We all have the same hearts, and our basic stories are the same," affirms Shaughnessy (1993, p. 105).

KEEPING CUSTOMERS FOR LIFE

A here-today, gone-tomorrow approach to healthcare customers no longer suffices. Be attuned to the seemingly insignificant things that make a tremendous impression on overall satisfaction and loyalty. "When my daughter was receiving radiation therapy at a clinic clear across the country," remembers Marianne, "a nurse arranged for a tutor to help her with her math at the Ronald McDonald House where we were staying. It made that nightmarish 6 weeks bearable, and helped to keep us focused on the future." Go the extra mile, and do it enthusiastically. Enthusiasm is a missing ingredient in so much of healthcare, yet it's a detail that really makes a difference.

If you want to keep customers for life, you can do it, say Cannie and Caplin (1991). But it can only be accomplished through people. If you take care of the people who take care of your customers, you take care of your customers. But you can be almost certain your customers are getting inferior service (and won't be happy) if:

- your people are unmotivated, disgruntled, or having a bad day;

- they are not trained or empowered to solve customers' problems or provide quality service;

- the boss treats them badly or otherwise devalues them;

- . . . managers model 'the customer is a pest'; or

- you make decisions and establish systems without considering the impact on your customers. (p. 5)

How do you keep customers for life? It's deceptively simple: "Find a need and fill it," as Norman Vincent Peale once said.

What Business Are We in?

Many issues facing healthcare today are psychological as well as financial. But one fundamental tenet is this: "Always know the answer to the question, 'What business are we in?'" (Moran, 1993). "I picked up my husband's shirts at the laundry the other day," says Mayme, a staff nurse, "and several buttons were cracked and broken on three of his best shirts. 'Don't worry,' the manager said with a smile. 'Buy some new buttons you like and we'll pick up the tab. We'll even sew them on for you.' That was all well and good, but that wasn't the service I thought I was purchasing from his company. It made me wonder how many times patients feel the same way about healthcare."

Customer-centered healthcare means that we tailor what a patient needs around their expectations and put them first (Rinaldo, 1986). Patients and families are the key to the success of any healthcare we deliver (Scott, 1993). "But nurses are often so rigid," a critical care nurse reflects. "Yet if you observe an episode where a nurse severs the strings of tradition, it can stay with you forever. One day, the ICU was hectic beyond belief, and the sister of one of our patients was digging in her pocket for change to buy a newspaper. In all of that chaos, my coworker stopped what she was doing and fed two quarters in the machine. She didn't say a word to me, and she didn't have to. Her actions said it all: the family is part of the patient."

Customer satisfaction can no longer be left to chance. "We will never cure our ailing healthcare system until our actions show that we care as much about people as we do processes," says Blancett (1992, p. 5). In other words, cater to your customers, and don't for a minute take your eyes off them. Patients *are* our work, not an interruption *to* our work. Success = quality and pride. We can't have one without the other. Ask yourself, "What is standing between me and my customer?" Then remember, what we need is all around us. Our combined expertise and wisdom are enough to meet the challenges we face as we look toward the future.

"With the many demands on a nurse's time, sometimes you have to stop for a minute and ask yourself: 'What could I be doing right now to be most effective?'" says Joan, a nurse in a psychiatric day care center. To be sure, that's a tall order. The well-known retailer, Stanley Marcus, had this to say about the long and tenuous road to satisfying customers: "There are only two things of importance. One is the customer, and the other is the product. If you take care of customers, they come back. If you take care of your product, it doesn't come back. It's just that simple. And it's just that difficult" (Whiteley, 1991, p. 211).

PARTNERS IN CARE

There's a growing discontent with fragmentation in healthcare that distresses both providers and patients. "At that clinic I take my mother to," says a waitress, "they're only concerned with body parts." Bernie Siegel, M.D. (1986) took a close look at the barriers which separated him from his patients and began encouraging them to address him by his first name. The change was well worth the risk, he says, as he now interacts person to person without the hindrance of a label.

Most of our healthcare delivery systems were designed during the industrial age. This is the information age. These days, many patients want to be partners in their care, and that calls for an entirely new approach. Still others hold fast to the traditional professional image of physician and nurse. "I used to love it when nurses came into my room wearing a crisp, white uniform, cap, and spotless shoes," recalls a great-grandmother. "It made me feel like I was in good hands."

A TEAM APPROACH

Consider what Donald Peterson, president of Ford Motor Company, said about the company's much touted comeback in the 1980's: "Customers are the focus of everything we do." Yet an equally important guiding principle for Ford was: "Employment involvement is our way of life. We are a team. We must treat each other with trust and respect" (Peterson & Hillkirk, 1991, p. 13).

Healthcare in the future will have to function as a team. "It used to be, if you wanted a job done right, you did it yourself," says a professor of nursing. "But today we must develop common goals despite our disparate backgrounds and philosophies. And we have to know that we'll support each other." How about this acronym for the word TEAM—Together Everyone Accomplishes More!

A RADICAL CHANGE IN THINKING

Ford Motor Company noticed that people are deeply concerned when a situation reaches crises proportions, and are generally open to trying new approaches to save their jobs. In these tumultuous days of healthcare reorganization, with talk of contracting out services to save facilities money and "replacing" registered nurses with less skilled personnel, the time is ripe for a change in thinking.

First it's crucial to realize that the financial problems facing healthcare are merely a symptom of a much deeper problem, a long chain of events that took years to create (Johnsson, 1990). As Crosby (1992, p. 136) says: "It has taken society a long time to realize that disasters ... don't just happen in one moment. They build up over time, and the clues are there for us to see." Any system left to its own devices will wear down. That's entropy, a basic law of physics.

The traditional approach to healthcare in America is broken, and it can't be fixed by working harder, cheaper, and faster ... strategies employed in the past. The antidote for this pocketbook pessimism is a patient-centered approach that designs care around the customer's needs, not those of the employee or organization. In one study of 311 hospital CEOs, 48% indicated that such a plan was already in the works (Sherer, 1994).

When confronted with change and uncertainty, the only thing persons can truly control is their attitude. Donna Thomas, Director of the Emergency Department at Primary Children's Medical Center in Salt Lake City, says: "To help my staff cope with the changes we were going through, I set up a workshop. It was the best thing I've done for them: the simple message that the only thing you can control is your attitude boosted their morale tremendously" (Hurley, 1994, p. 35).

When something was broken in the past, we used to put a little money on the problem. That doesn't work anymore. We must look closely at the root cause of problems and not just symptoms. "In many ways, the changes we're witnessing in healthcare are like a funeral," says Kay, a perinatal nurse. "We must grieve the loss of 'the way things used to be.'"

A Backward Glance

Photographer Rob Karosis travels the grounds of American resorts with his vintage wood, leather, and brass camera in tow. His mission? Karosis snaps photographs that could easily be mistaken for those taken 50 years before. There are moments when the past and present seem to merge, he contends, and his impressive work has earned him a place in Polaroid's permanent collection. While some things have, of course, changed drastically, many details—massive columns; stately, hand-carved staircases; rolling, carpeted grounds; adirondack porch chairs—are timeless in their appeal. Oh, the insight of hindsight!

Sometimes by looking back, we notice that the basics haven't really changed at all. That idea certainly holds water in the area of customer satisfaction. If we, like Karosis, were to photograph patients in the 1990's and compare their basic human needs with those of even a century ago, I think we'd be surprised. Even with the explosion of technology, it's still the personalized details—sincere caring, service, respect—that engender a feeling of trust. While it's important to study the past, we must manage the future.

FIND YOUR SERVICE NICHE

In a speech to the Second Presbyterian Church of Springfield, Illinois, on February 2, 1842, Abraham Lincoln said:

> It is an old and true maxim that a drop of honey catches more flies than a gallon of gall. So with men. If you would win a man to your cause, first convince him that you are his sincere friend. Therein is a drop of honey that catches his heart, which, say what he will, is the great high road to his reason, and which, once gained, you will find but little trouble in convincing his judgement of the justice of your cause, if indeed that cause really be a just one.

Service is the way to catch today's consumer with honey. Many healthcare organizations are selling the same products; it's service that distinguishes the good from the better and the better from the best. To give your organization the competitive edge, discover your service niche. It's not business as usual anymore. Better to do a limited number of things well than to try your hand at everything coming down the pike. Poor service is simply not cost effective (Lathrop, 1993).

Waste not, Want not

Customers in all realms of society are environmentally conscious and are concerned about undue waste. Explore cost containment strategies in your organization, perhaps via a cost awareness fair. Ask staff for insight on ways to cut waste in both material and human resources. And remember, nothing is more wasteful than doing something which shouldn't be done at all.

Changing Customer Needs

Take a trip down memory lane and look back at the Ford Motor Company. Henry Ford's pronouncement that the customer "could have any color so long as it was black" became a classic example of the incorrect response to changing customer needs (Tucker, 1991, p. 86). Customer-centered care means customizing healthcare to the customer's needs. Just as General Motors hit upon the idea of a "car for every purse and purpose" (Tucker, 1991, p. 86), healthcare must also respond to ever-changing expectations. "Satisfaction used to be something that validated the way we did business," observes Greg Lea. "Now it drives it. That is a dramatic change" (George & Weimerskirch, 1994, p. 33). Choice and change are the bywords of the 1990's.

In industry, companies who succeed are the ones who understand the changing needs of their customers. Remember the trend in the 1950's and 1960's of door-to-door Avon sales representatives? Women stayed at home in those days, and security was less of a threat. "Avon Calling" was a welcome break from the mundane chores of homemaking. Today's woman, however, typically works outside the home and wouldn't open her door to a stranger if she were home. In response to the customer's changing needs, Avon began marketing products to the working woman with great success. Having a quality product isn't enough; you have to put your customer in the picture.

Willingham (1992) makes the all-important distinction that we aren't in business to deliver products or services, but rather to provide the benefits of those products or services to people. Let's say you offer a superb pulmonary fitness program at your facility. You don't sell your lung program. You sell what the program can do for your patients. They can get a program just about anywhere. What they want to know is how your program is going to help them.

THE AGING AMERICAN PUBLIC

The fastest growing segment of the American population is the elderly. Since 1990, the percentage of Americans age 65 and older has tripled, and the older population in general is getting older. It's estimated that by the year 2030, there will be approximately 70 million older Americans, comprising 20% of the population (AARP, 1993).

THE CHANGING AMERICAN HEALTHCARE WORKER

Woody Allen once mused that 80% of success in life is showing up. All jokes aside, the American work ethic, like other traditional values, is being reevaluated (Colson & Eckerd, 1991; Gordon, 1991; Cheney, 1993). Many factors come into play: a growing recognition that workaholism is unhealthy, a distrustful work force, and a feeling of exploitation among dedicated workers who have given their all, only to find themselves forgotten when their place of employment shuts down. This is a "911" symbol for healthcare and customer satisfaction.

"The loss of the work ethic," contend Colson and Eckerd (1991, p. 1), "does not begin in the workplace; it begins in the hearts of people—in the values that motivate them or fail to motivate them."

One nurse who freelances as an artist suggests that what is needed is a change in attitude, to encompass the mindset of a freelancer who "gets rewarded commensurate with the job accomplished. If my art work isn't up to snuff, it doesn't sell out in the marketplace," she says. "But on the other hand, that makes me take great pride in what I do."

"I do precious little some days at work any more," a 30-year veteran of the nursing profession admits reluctantly. "I'm the first to say, "I'm nowhere near excellence. The fire is gone. I do the absolute minimum to get by.'"

In healthcare, workers commonly cite that administration is insensitive or unaware of the problems of front-line workers. But first and foremost, work must have meaning. "When you are able to see how your job benefits your customers," says Scott (1991, p. 2), "your personal satisfaction goes up. You add meaning to your work when you have a clear customer orientation."

Techniques such as threats, intimidation, and fear may be productive in the short term, but will never permanently motivate an employee, especially in these changing times. Nor do job security, improved working conditions, and financial compensation top the list. There is a surprising "perception gap" between what workers really want and what top administration assumes they want (Twentier, 1994). Feedback, respect, recognition, and improved employer-employee relations are most important. If you want staff to care about your business, you must get to the heart of the matter.

In any business, quality can't happen in the absence of a competent, dedicated work force. It's people who play the biggest role in customer satisfaction, but they must be empowered to do so. "Make it your business to take care of your people, and your people will take care of you" (Twentier, 1994, p. 60).

BE INNOVATIVE

Perhaps the staff in your organization have a non-traditional or even slightly "off the wall" idea for improving service or care that your customers haven't articulated. The solution? Consider it. An example of this strategy is found in the archives of Kodak. A meager 5% of their customers identified the need for expedient photo processing. Then 1-hour processing centers became all the rage, and the rest is history (Tucker, 1991, p. 38). Sometimes customers don't know exactly what they want until they see it.

One hospital came up with the idea of drive-thru flu vaccines. Consumers who had never imagined such a concept loved it. The booming business earned a spot in the local paper and on the evening news, which resulted in prime-time patient education as well as further advertisement for the facility. With an average of 4 out of 10 hospital beds empty in this country, innovative and effective marketing is all the more important (Inlander & Weiner, 1993). Be creative and let your imagination soar. Go with your hunches and, like this hospital, you just may find you're king of the road.

What Is Your Vision?

Vision is a key to success, whether it be with individuals or with organizations. Comments Philip B. Crosby (1992, p. 197), a leader in America's quality revolution: "Reading the autobiographies and biographies of successful people shows us that most of them had a clear vision of what they wanted their lives to be."

It's advice as ancient as The Bible, which says: "Where there is no vision, the people perish" (Proverbs 29:18). One of the most important statements in any organization is the vision statement, because it articulates, in a nutshell, the future of that organization.

Ray Kroc, the founder of McDonald's, stated his vision like this: "Quality, Service, Cleanliness, Value" (Whiteley, 1991). Federal Express's vision statement, based on the philosophy of PEOPLE-SERVICE-PROFIT, delivers what it promises, and was the first major service company to receive the prestigious Malcolm Baldridge National Quality Award.

"We can no longer stand on the sidelines and react to what happens," stresses a public health nurse. "We must be prepared and perceptive even to the subtle changes in healthcare."

Take Your Service to the Customer

The other day I overheard a patient remark on a hospital elevator, "They run you here and there . . . to X-ray . . . the lab . . . it aggravates me to no end." Have you ever noticed the accommodating approach of veterinarians when dealing with their customers? The pet is typically brought to an examining area where its blood is drawn, X-rays are taken, medications are administered, and prescriptions refilled—all in one general area. They bring their care right to the customer.

I didn't think that sort of thing ever happened to people, but I was wrong. One winter I had a root canal and experienced some complications on Super Bowl Sunday, of all days. In excruciating pain, I was still very hesitant to call my dentist's answering service. To my surprise, the call I made was returned within 30 minutes, and there was never any doubt he would see me at my convenience. When I asked him why he dropped everything to check on me, he replied: "My family ran an auto parts store when I was growing up, and we always opened up on Sunday when someone needed something." It was one of life's "Aha!" moments and a great example of how healthcare could change its paradigm to reexamine the way we do our day-to-day business.

Ruth relates another story: "My 5-year-old son had stuck his hand through a glass door and I took him to a clinic to have it checked out. He was so upset that the nurse practitioner examined him in the waiting room on his own terms. What would have been an hour of kicking and screaming didn't happen because of her sensitivity."

The Trend Toward Complementary Therapies

Healthcare consumers are becoming increasingly interested in complementary (sometimes called alternative) types of therapy as an adjunct to modern technological medicine. These range from massage therapy to meditation to therapeutic touch to acupuncture. "No longer are such modalities pursued solely by metaphysicians and parapsychologists," remarks a psychiatric clinical nurse specialist, "but by those in traditional healthcare roles as well. Many of these techniques appeal to the emotional and spiritual aspects of a person, inadequately addressed by our technology-based healthcare system which so often doesn't reach the human, personal part of us."

Technology, as wondrous as it can be, simply can't satisfy the cravings of the human spirit. Many "traditional" caregivers are recognizing the limitations of modern healthcare as we know it. Says one family practice physician: "If patients tell me that carrying a watermelon under their left arm makes them feel better, I say, 'Carry that watermelon' (within limits, of course). Who am I to discount what's working?"

As the System Evolves

Most Americans agree that the healthcare system needs to change—they just aren't sure how. Regardless of what happens over the next two decades, it is likely to be painful for everyone: consumers, payers, employers, and clinicians (Brown, Nelson, Bronkesh, & Wood, 1993). The ultimate goal is improved quality and access to care at less expense (Whyte & Beall, 1995). In a system of true healthcare reform, managed care organizations, healthcare professionals, and pharmaceutical companies will work together to understand and enhance the clinical decision-making process, and measurably improve the quality and continuity of care (Forster, 1995).

"I divide the world into three classes," said Nicholas Murray Butler, "the few who make things happen, the many who watch things happen, and the overwhelming majority who have no notion of what happened." As we approach a future of unprecedented change, competitiveness, and uncertainty, let's find ourselves among those healthcare providers who make the best things happen. For if we don't satisfy our customers, someone else most assuredly will.

References

AARP. (1993). *A profile of older Americans.* AARP.

Barnes, D., Eribes, C., Juarbe, T., Nelson, M., Proctor, S., Sawyer, L., Shaul, M., & Meleis, A. I. (1995). Primary health care and primary care: A confusion of philosophies. *Nursing Outlook, 43*(1), 7-16.

Berwick, D. M., Godfrey, A. B., & Roessner, J. (1990). *Curing health care* (p. 159-165). San Francisco: Jossey-Bass, Inc.

Blancett, S. S. (1992). Satisfaction: It's more than effectiveness and efficiency. *Journal of Nursing Administration, 22*(2), 5.

Brown, S. W., Nelson, A., & Bronkesh, S. J., & Wood, S. D. (1993). *Patient satisfaction pays: Quality service for practice success.* Gaithersburg, MD: Aspen Publishers, Inc.

Cannie, J. K., & Caplin, D. (1991). *Keeping customers for life.* New York: AMACOM.

Cheney, L. (1993, April 6). What ever happened to hard work? *The Wall Street Journal.*

Clements, M. (1993, Feb. 28). The growing crisis in healthcare. *Parade: The Sunday Oregonian,* 4.

Colson, C., & Eckerd, J. (1991). *Why America doesn't work.* Dallas: Word Publishing.

Crosby, P. B. (1992). *Completeness: Quality for the 21st century.* New York: Penguin Books USA, Inc.

Doyle, E. (1995). Tools to help internists deliver more preventive care. *American College of Physicians, 15*(4), 4-5.

Flynn, A. M., & Kilgallen, M. E. (1993). Case management: A multidisciplinary approach to the evaluation of cost and quality standards. *Journal of Nursing Care Quality, 8*(1), 58-66.

Forster, J. (1995). Disease management in 1995. *Patient Care, 29*(8), 7.

Gatty, B. (1993). Health system reform: The sudden shift toward primary care. *Geriatrics, 48*(11), 78-82.

George, S., & Weimerskirch, A. (1994). *Total quality management: Strategies and techniques proven at today's most successful companies.* New York: John Wiley and Sons, Inc.

Gordon, S. J. (1991, Nov. 5). Work ethics. *Family Circle,* 176.

Gray, Y. L., & Bailey, N. C. (1995). Cluster care: An alternative to traditional care. *Home Healthcare Nurse, 13*(2), 41-44.

Hurley, M. L. (1994). Where will you work tomorrow? *RN, 57*(8), 31-35.

Inlander, C. B., & Weiner, E. (1993). *Take this book to the hospital with you.* New Jersey: Wings Books.

Johnson, E. A. (1995). The public's future perspective on managed care. *Health Care Management Review, 20*(2), 45-47.

Johnsson, J. (1990, Sept. 5). Investors link quality of care to the bottom line. *Hospitals,* 86.

Kupecz, D. B. (1994, August). The nurse practitioner movement in the VA. *V.A. Practitioner,* 29-33.

Lansky, D. (1995). Health care quality: All dressed up with nowhere to go. *Journal of Quality Improvement, 21*(1), 32-33.

Mack, J. L., File, K. M., Horwitz, J. E., & Prince, R. A. (1995). The effect of urgency on patient satisfaction and future emergency department choice. *Health Care Management Review, 20*(2), 7-15.

Meissner, J. E., & Carey, K. W. (1994). How's your job security? *Nursing 94, 24*(7), 33-38.

Moran, R. A. (1993). *Never confuse a memo with reality (and other business lessons too simple not to know).* New York: Harper Collins Publishers.

Moyers, B. (1993). *Healing and the mind.* New York: Doubleday.

Nelson, E. C., Rust, R. T., Zahorik, A., Rose, R. L., Batalden, P., & Siemanski, B. A. (1992). Do patient perceptions of quality relate to hospital financial performance? *Journal of Health Care Marketing, 12,* 6-13.

Peterson, D. E., & Hillkirk, J. (1991). *A better idea: Redefining the way Americans work.* Boston: Houghton Mifflin Co.

Press, I., Ganey, R. F., & Malone, M. P. (1991, Feb.). Satisfied patients can spell financial well-being. *Healthcare Financial Management,* 34-42.

Rinaldo, D. G. (1986). Our patients still need tender loving care. *RN, 49*(10), 67.

RN News Watch. (1994a). Home care growth is a sure bet, if insurers go along. *RN, 57*(6), 14.

RN News Watch. (1994b). A new nursing curriculum is a sign of the times. *RN, 57*(4), 15.

Schiff, R. L., Goldberg, D., & Ansell, D. A. (1992). Access to health care. In R.P. Wenzel (Ed.), *Assessing quality health care* (pp. 139-155). Baltimore: Williams & Wilkins.

Scott, D. (1991). *Customer satisfaction: The other half of your job.* Menlo Park, CA: Crisp Publications, Inc.

Scott, L. (1993). *It's a dog's world.* Carlsbad, CA: CRM Films Leaders Guide.

Shaughnessy, S. (1993). *Walking on alligators: A book of meditations for writers.* New York: Harper Collins Publishers.

Sherer, J. L. (1994, March). Putting patients first. *Trustee,* 14-16.

Sherman, V. C. (1993). *Creating the new American hospital: A time for greatness.* San Francisco: Jossey-Bass, Inc.

Shortell, S. M. (1995, June). The future of hospitals and health care management. *FORUM: VA Health Services Research and Development*, 1-3.

Siegel, B. S. (1986). *Love, medicine and miracles.* New York: Harper & Row Publishers, Inc.

Tucker, R. B. (1991). *Managing the future.* New York: G.P. Putnam's Sons.

Twentier, J. D. (1994). *The positive power of praising people.* Nashville: Thomas, Nelson, Inc.

Warner, R. R. (1992). Nurses' empathy and patients' satisfaction with nursing care. *Journal of the New York State Nurses' Association, 23*(4), 8-11.

Whiteley, R. C. (1991). *The customer driven company: Moving from talk to action.* Reading, MA: Addison-Wesley Publishing Co.

Whyte, J. J., & Beall, D. P. (1995). A physician's freedom to choose. *Journal of the American Medical Association, 273*(16), 1238a.

Willingham, R. (1992). *Hey I'm the customer.* Englewood Cliffs, NJ: Prentice Hall.

Zanca, J. A. (1995). Home health: The ultimate in care. *Cancer Nursing News, 13*(1), 1, 5.

Chapter 3

QUALITY ISN'T A COINCIDENCE

We shall build good ships here.
At a profit if we can.
At a loss if we must.
But always good ships.

— Collis P. Huntington, founder,
Newport News Shipbuilding and Dry Dock Company, 1886

H ealthcare organizations are aptly turning to the corporate world for many valuable lessons about quality and customer satisfaction. Here's what some of them have to say:

- Motorola: "Quality is not an assignable task. It must be rooted and institutionalized in every process. It is everyone's responsibility" (George & Weimerskirch, 1994, p. 79).

- Satisfaction Guaranteed Eateries: "Always deal with complaints before they're made" (Whiteley, 1991, p. 1).

- Rubbermaid: "Our customers are not there to field-test our products" (Tucker, 1991, p. 198).

- T.J. Maxx: "The maxx for the minimum."

- DeMet's Chocolate Factory: " ... We're always raising our own standard of excellence."

- Ford Motor Company: "The quality continues."

- W.M. Green & Company: "Offer exceptional merchandise to thousands of customers through the convenience of catalog shopping, yet serve each customer one at a time."

- L.L. Bean: "Service is just a day-in, day-out, ongoing, never-ending, persevering, compassionate type of activity" (Brown, Nelson, Bronkesh, & Wood, 1993, p. 290).

- Zenith: "Quality goes in before the name goes on."

I recently received a catalog from a mail-order company that featured a cartoon in which a clerk and a customer were having a discussion about quality. "Just so you understand in advance," the tongue-in-cheek caption read, "we're not old-time craftsmen, and we don't take pride in our work." *That's precisely what healthcare customers are after,* I thought. *They want the pride and down-home personalization of the past, combined with the best of today's technology.* And if there's anything the changes in healthcare are teaching us, it's when you're out of quality, you're out of business. But quality doesn't just happen, especially in a budget-cutting environment. Rather, it is the result of careful planning and a commitment to excellence, despite reductions in resources.

JUST WHAT IS QUALITY?

What is quality? I posed that question to a group of nurses and here's what I heard:

- "Quality is having the desired clinical outcome."

- "Quality is giving patients the kind of care you'd give to your own loved one."

- "Quality is when a patient leaves your facility and brags of the care they received."

- "Quality is being the best you can be."

- And some of the best advice from the world of health-care is found in a motto of the American Red Cross: "Quality saves lives."

How Do the Experts Define Quality?

- Webster (Merriam Webster, Inc., 1991, p. 963): "1.) Degree of excellence; 2.) Superiority in kind; 3.) A distinguishing attribute."

- Philip B. Crosby (1992, flyleaf): "Quality is the skeletal structure of an organization."

- Joseph Juran (The National Association of Quality Assurance Professionals, 1991, pp. 7–8): "Quality is product performance that results in customer satisfaction and freedom from product deficiencies that avoid customer dissatisfaction."

- The Joint Commission on Accreditation of Healthcare Organizations (JCAHO) (1994, p. 181): "The degree to which health services for individuals and populations increase the likelihood of desired health outcomes and are consistent with current professional knowledge."

Healthcare Quality: A Historical Perspective

In 1916, Codman observed:

> I'm called eccentric for saying that hospitals must find out what their results are; must analyze their results to find their strong and weak points; to care for what cases they can

> care for well; must assign staff, for better reasons than
> seniority, the calendar of convenience; must promote staff
> on what they can and do accomplish—such opinions will not
> be eccentric a few years hence.

As early as 1918, standards for hospitals were published by the American College of Surgeons, the forerunner of the JCAHO. In 1951, the JCAHO was formally established, and since 1966, the U.S. government has depended on them to determine eligibility of healthcare organizations for Medicare and Medicaid reimbursement (Joint Commission Perspectives, 1994).

THE ACCREDITATION PROCESS

Any U.S. healthcare organization may apply for a JCAHO accreditation survey as long as there are applicable standards for that organization. In addition to accrediting hospitals, JCAHO also has standards for non-hospital-based psychiatric and substance abuse organizations such as community mental health centers, as well as long-term care facilities, home and ambulatory care organizations, organization-based pathology and clinical laboratory services, and other healthcare networks (JCAHO, 1994). Similar organizations are judged by identical criteria.

An accreditation survey lasts 3 to 5 days, with accreditation granted for 3 years. Categories of accreditation are: accreditation with commendation, accreditation, conditional accreditation, provisional accreditation, and not accredited. If an organization is found to have deficiencies that require a focused survey zeroing in on one or more areas of concern, this will generally be scheduled within 6 months of the initial survey. In addition, a 5% random sample of accredited organizations now undergoes an unannounced mid-cycle survey which focuses on performance areas identified as being problematic nationwide within the past year (JCAHO, 1994).

The JCAHO has begun disclosing accreditation performance information about individual facilities to the public (Ente, 1994), including the agency's overall score, how that score compares to other facilities, and recommendations for improvement. While JCAHO accreditation doesn't address specific patient outcomes, an institution's accreditation score is a good predictor of them. JCAHO standards represent the recognized standard for healthcare organizations. In the future, this will likely be a marketing tool to aid healthcare facilities in securing managed care, insurance, and other contracts (Bowers, Swan, & Koehler, 1994; Greene, 1995), and patients themselves in choosing providers of care.

While JCAHO is the accreditation body most strongly having impact on U.S. healthcare organizations, your facility may be subject to other site visits. Community Health Accreditation Program, Inc. (CHAP), for example, is a consumer-driven accreditation body which sets quality standards for organizations that provide home healthcare. Originally a division of the National League for Nursing, CHAP is the only accrediting body that has established outcome measures of quality for home healthcare, and is highly attuned to customer satisfaction. It advises consumers to ascertain that the agency they're considering for home healthcare regularly solicits input from patients (CHAP, 1995).

Once, while he was hoeing his garden, someone asked St. Francis of Assisi what he would do if he were to learn that he would die that evening before sunset. His answer? "I would finish hoeing my garden." That's appropriate advice for healthcare agencies at any point in their accreditation cycle.

In the past, people tended to kick into gear and flex their quality muscles with the news that an accreditation agency was on the way, then breathe a collective sigh of relief when they left. When an institution received reaccreditation, some employees had the mistaken notion that they could "stop hoeing" for another few years. "Let's get this quality stuff over with so we can get back to our 'real' jobs," as one hospital staff member put it. But not so anymore.

"Thankfully, we're getting away from saying we do this and that because JCAHO says to do it," observes a vice president for nursing. "We do things because it's good business, and we want to continue to improve the care we provide. Accreditation should merely be a reflection of that process." Today, JCAHO's standards are more patient-centered than ever, instructing facilities to address actual performance, not merely the capacity for that performance.

In the past, a large segment of a JCAHO survey was conducted in an office setting where managers produced reams of policies and procedures. These days, however, surveyors spend the majority of their time in patient care areas assessing the bottom line: Does the care provided make a difference for customers? Are institutions doing the right things and doing them well? Are organizations structured to improve the outcomes of patient care? Are patients satisfied with their care? Are facilities wasting precious resources because of unnecessary duplication of activities? Are organizations addressing the intent of the standards in a manner which best meets the unique needs of their patient population?

Facilities are now assessed across the entire organization rather than as separate departments. "There is simply no such thing as 'Nursing QA' anymore," reflects a quality manager. "We have to demonstrate that we all really work together to improve the quality of care, not just on paper." Indeed, it's impossible for one service in an institution to "carry the hospital" during a JCAHO survey because facilities are judged as a complete entity in their efforts to improve organizational performance.

JCAHO DIMENSIONS OF QUALITY

When it comes to evaluating healthcare, quality boils down to doing the right things right. But what is important to measure? The JCAHO (1994) has identified nine dimensions of quality that can determine how a healthcare organization's functions may affect patients. They fall into two categories: doing the right thing and doing the right thing well, discussed below with selected clinical examples.

Doing the Right Thing

1. Efficacy: Did the care or intervention achieve the desired or anticipated outcome? If a patient is enrolled in a clinical trial for a new antihypertensive medication, for instance, did he or she achieve the desired clinical response?

2. Appropriateness: Is the care or intervention provided relevant to and appropriate for the patient's clinical need? Here's an example of when interventions weren't appropriate because of an inaccurate preoperative assessment. During her preoperative workup, a patient completed a self-assessment to alert the anesthesia staff of risk factors. When the computer posed the question, "Have you ever smoked, and if so, how much?" the patient entered "Yes," and "Two packages." The computer jumped to the next question without giving the patient the opportunity to explain that she had only smoked two packages of cigarettes in her entire life.

    Assuming the response meant the patient had smoked two packages per day, the anesthesia staff ordered an expensive pulmonary workup and postoperative respiratory therapy treatments which were inappropriate for the patient's clinical needs. This could have been avoided by clarifying information with the patient, relating to her as a human being and not merely a computer response.

Doing the Right Thing Well

3. Availability: Is the service or product available to meet the patient's need? If a hospital cares for patients who have suffered a cerebrovascular accident, for instance, are there adequate rehabilitation and prosthetic resources? Does that rural patient, newly diagnosed with cancer, have access to the radiation therapy required for state-of-the-art treatment?

4. Timeliness: Is the care or intervention provided to the patient at the most beneficial time? Here's a not-so-funny real experience that emphasizes the importance of timeliness. A patient with asthma had an aminophylline level drawn just prior to her hospital discharge. Several days later, a frantic secretary telephoned the patient's mother with the message that "her daugh-

ter's level was way off and her medication dosage needed to be changed—quick!" When the mother asked
when she should bring her daughter in for follow-up,
the secretary skimmed the scheduling book and replied,
"How about a week from Friday?"

How long do patients wait in your prenatal clinic? What
is your OR cancellation rate due to failure to obtain
medical clearance in time for a scheduled surgical procedure? Doing something right the first time (such as
correctly collecting a specimen so it doesn't have to be
repeated and therapy delayed) is also an important
timeliness issue. Time is money to healthcare organizations, and it's money to customers who experience
excessive delays.

5. Effectiveness: Is the care or intervention provided in the
    correct manner, given the current state of knowledge?
    Your medical center may utilize several approved treat-
    ment modalities for pressure ulcers. Clinical trials may
    have shown all of them to be efficacious, and you may
    follow the manufacturer's directions to the letter in
    using a particular product. But the question remains,
    "Does it produce the desired clinical outcome in an indi-
    vidual patient—does it really work?" If it doesn't, it isn't
    effective, plain and simple.

6. Continuity: Is the care or intervention provided for the
    patient coordinated over time, with respect to other ser-
    vices and providers? Did patient education and dis-
    charge planning involve all appropriate members of the
    interdisciplinary team as well as family and community
    support systems? Were appropriate referrals initiated to
    ensure that quality of care is uninterrupted post-dis-
    charge?

    Since nursing is often the vital link in continuity of care
    (and is the 24-hour continuity for hospitals), the illus-
    trations for this dimension of quality are numerous.
    When departments in your healthcare agency don't

cooperate with one another, it's time to put your heads together to take a close look at how you do business. Then use that information to improve quality of care, not make counterproductive judgment calls about "those other departments."

7. Safety: Are the risks of procedures and interventions, as well as the hospital environment, kept to a minimum for patients, visitors, and healthcare workers? Are current Centers for Disease Control (CDC) and Occupational Safety and Health Administration (OSHA) recommendations followed? Are these communicated to external customers via patient/family education and to staff via ongoing inservice education? Are patients assessed on admission and throughout hospitalization, as appropriate, to determine if they are at increased risk for falls, nosocomial infection, pressure ulcers, and other pertinent incidents?

8. Efficiency: Is there a clear relationship between outcomes of care and resources allocated to deliver that care? If nursing care is provided via a primary nursing model, is this the best utilization of resources given the mix of your non-professional and professional staff? Do patients complain that "fifteen different people asked me the same questions when I was admitted"? These are but two examples of efficiency issues.

9. Respect and Caring: Are patients and their families involved in decisions related to their care? Are personnel sensitive and respectful, giving consideration to individual differences? Is a sincere attempt made to get to know the patient rather than assuming "He's just like the rest of those elderly patients"? In the delivery of healthcare, quality, from the customer's viewpoint, has as much to do with perception as with the actual product. Although this dimension of quality is less tangible than the previous eight, it's one of the most crucial for customer satisfaction.

HOW CONSUMERS DEFINE QUALITY

Customer satisfaction is the yardstick by which consumer perceptions of quality are defined. What quality was to the 1980's, customer satisfaction will be to the 1990's.

Study the advertisements in consumer publications, and you'll gain a renewed appreciation for what customers want and expect in healthcare. A Ford Motor Company ad, for example, emphasizes the importance of listening to your customers. "It's part of the learning process that leads to quality," it says.

General Motors asserts in one of their advertisements that "Sometimes responding to customer input means scrapping a beloved notion . . . the customer isn't just somebody with an opinion. The customer is a colleague with a whole lot of clout."

Or how about a Revlon Cosmetics ad campaign that alerts potential customers to the "measurable results" of its new night cream?

A guarantee establishes a standard for a product or service, and places the focus where it belongs—on the customer. Let's say a mail-order establishment promises that your money will be cheerfully refunded at any time and for any reason. Both the clerk and the customer then share a common frame of reference and expectation for both the quality of the product and the service.

But in healthcare there are no guarantees, and all too often providers and patients don't share a common reference point. Rather, healthcare consumers often equate the quality of care they receive with the quality of staff interpersonal skills. While they are understandably weary of empty slogans and fail-to-deliver promises, research shows a strong relationship between effective communication and overall patient satisfaction (Hall, Roter, & Katz, 1988).

A study measuring adolescents' satisfaction with nursing care found that while teens were most satisfied with the technical aspects of their care, they were least satisfied with the interpersonal dimension (Turner & Matthews, 1991). In a study of medical-surgical patients, Bader (1988) found that patient satisfaction was less in the affective dimension of nursing practice. She concluded that satisfaction with nursing care would increase if more emphasis was placed on addressing emotional needs of patients.

Healthcare customers' expectations are also fueled by the media, and competition and survival of any organization is related to price and perceived quality of service and care (Berwick, Blanton, & Roessner, 1990). "Good things aren't cheap and cheap things aren't good," contends one customer. It's a paraphrase on the old adage that you get what you pay for. Yet when quality is in clear focus—in healthcare and in business—costs decrease because of less rework, fewer mistakes and delays, and more effective use of people, time, and materials. Our grandmothers' generation had a wonderful philosophy that bears a heavy load of truth today: Do it right the first time.

While today's healthcare customer may respect our education and expertise, they expect measurable performance, not merely platitudes. Good enough is no longer good enough. Maintaining the status quo spells death for today's healthcare organizations. Getting it right 99.9% of the time, to cite three examples, is the equivalent of two daily unsafe landings at O'Hare International Airport, 12 babies given to the wrong parents each day, and 20,000 incorrect prescriptions written over a 1-year period (Berglund, 1994). In healthcare we used to talk in terms of thresholds, and many were set at 95% compliance. But if we say it's okay to meet expectations only 95% of the time, we're sending out a powerful negative message in the way we approach our customers.

Quality doesn't happen without careful planning and attention to details. Consider this definition of quality posted in the lobby of a large outpatient clinic: "Quality is never an accident; it is always the result of high intention, sincere effort, intelligent direction and skillful execution; it represents the wise choice of many alternatives."

THE TWO SIDES OF QUALITY

There are two sides of healthcare quality: the clinical dimension (or how we define it) and the caring dimension (or how our customers define it). Neither dimension spells quality in the absence of the other (Koska, 1989). Sure, it's important that we have the latest equipment and a pleasing physical facility, but customers judge our reliability, our responsiveness, and our empathy as well, even though these intangible aspects are much more difficult to measure.

When over 600 hospital CEOs were asked to define the most significant factors in providing high-quality care, nursing care, not surprisingly, topped the list of 10 choices: 97.3% as opposed to 89.9% for state-of-the-art technology (Koska, 1989). But in today's healthcare milieu, quality must also be quantifiable and consider the highly variable expectations, perceptions, and standards of both internal and external customers. This includes virtually everyone: patients, families, caregivers, third-party payers, suppliers, and outside accreditation bodies (The National Association of Healthcare Professionals, 1991).

CUSTOMER PERCEPTIONS

In order to survive, healthcare organizations must move from the outdated quality assurance mode to improving quality from the viewpoint of customers. Quality service means "the ability to meet customers' requirements" (Cannie & Caplin, 1991, p. 113). In other words, designing healthcare around the customer's—not the provider's—needs.

"Well, we make things right if a patient or family member is unsatisfied," you might argue. But while a good backup plan is commendable, it's likely a source of irritation in the customer's mind. As Crosby (1992, p. 20) points out, "The customer will remember the problem and inconvenience long after they have forgotten the effectiveness of the repair."

Remember, every job has to stand alone. Don't settle for mediocrity. Customers are looking for uncompromising quality. The old adage, "Don't do things too bad or too good" won't work today. There's nothing in the middle of the road except yellow lines and dead opossums.

A patient really doesn't care what the JCAHO manual says about quality or whether an I.V. is administered by an R.N. or L.P.N. Patients perceive quality in the context of their own experience (Omachonu, 1990). They simply want to feel they are receiving high-quality care, and any deviation from this expectation can leave them with a lasting negative perception of the entire experience.

THE MANY NAMES OF QUALITY

You've probably heard quality described in various (and often confusing) buzzwords and synonyms through the years. QA (or Quality Assurance) was the earlier terminology and was a reactive, service-specific, fragmented approach which focused on "putting out fires" and "finding bad apples" in an organization through the maddening monotony of "audits." While QA had many positive aspects, it was all too often viewed as punitive and associated with "a paper program" that failed to make any lasting difference. In addition, it did not merge the cooperative efforts of staff from different departments to address a shared problem.

In recent years, the terminology evolved to QM (Quality Management) or QAI (Quality Assessment and Improvement). More recently, CQI (Continuous Quality Improvement), which uses the concepts of TQM (Total Quality Management), as piloted in industry, has come into vogue in healthcare.

CONTINUOUS QUALITY IMPROVEMENT

While all of these terms may seem to be one and the same, in actuality they are as different as "lightening and the lightning bug," as Mark Twain would have said. Terms used to define quality in times past are vastly more limiting than the newer CQI approach (Crosby, 1992, p. xv). The English language lacks a single word to express the idea of continuously improving quality (Brown et al., 1993). The Japanese, however, well-schooled in the concept at long last adopted by America, have a word for it: "kaizan."

While terminology varies from facility to facility, CQI is a proactive approach which recognizes that the majority of problems in an institution are related to a system's inefficiency, rather than to individual employees. This lessens defensiveness of staff (Ziegenfuss & O'Rourke, 1995), decreases costly duplication efforts, and promotes an atmosphere of employee empowerment conducive to risk-taking and meeting customer needs.

CQI and the JCAHO acknowledge that the processes of an organization are the key determinants in providing efficient and effective care translating into optimal clinical outcomes. Aimed at prevention and timely intervention, they are centered on the identified needs of customers. A guiding philosophy is using customer input to improve organizational performance. As Deming (1986) and others (Moore & Moore, 1993) have asserted, organizations which will experience long-term success will be those who are able to meet and exceed the needs and expectations of their customers.

Because processes in healthcare always involve people, there is always an opportunity to improve care and services. By building on the lessons learned in traditional QA, CQI necessitates that all employees (from the leadership to the front-line staff) adopt the idea that quality is everyone's responsibility, not merely a select few who may work in the "Quality" department.

CQI focuses on systems and major processes, such as Education, Assessment of Patients, and Patient Rights and Organizational Ethics. It is dependent on hard statistical data (management by fact rather than anecdotes or gut feelings) for decision making. "The question we must always be asking ourselves is 'What does the data have to do with patient care and their ultimate satisfaction with the care they receive?'" emphasizes a CQI facilitator. Nurses are at an obvious advantage with CQI because it builds on the familiar concept of the nursing process.

A study of 3,000 hospitals indicated that 69% were utilizing the CQI philosophy to improve quality of care. While a number of approaches were cited, the majority of those surveyed indicated that they had incorporated the tenets of quality gurus: W. Edwards Deming, Joseph Juran, or Philip Crosby (Haddock, Nosky, Fargason, & Kurz, 1995). While the JCAHO doesn't mandate a spe-

cific approach to ensuring quality, a CQI model is highly congruent with accreditation standards (JCAHO, 1994).

Staff education and leadership commitment are critical factors
to successful implementation of CQI, as is the culture of the organization. According to one study of 61 hospitals, those with a group
development-oriented culture fared better than those with layers of
red tape and bureaucracy (Shortell, 1995). "We're trying to restruc-
ture the environment through the use of teams and the effective
distribution of responsibility," said one hospital president and
CEO. "We're trying to get away from the traditional organizational
structure that fostered territorialism and inhibited communication" (Staff, 1993, p. 17).

CQI is not a superficial quick fix, but rather a means to a more
permanent solution for an identified problem. It is simple and
focused, rather than complex and grandiose. Rather than trying to
solve all of an organization's problems in one fell swoop, you break
issues down to one point in the process where you can identify a
clear-cut problem. Once you solve that problem, you tackle another.

If an organization isn't truly committed to the slow but sure
process of interdisciplinary collaboration, discouragement can easily set in. "CQI reminds me of the early days of my mortgage,"
muses a unit manager. "We were paying the same house payment
back then, but it took awhile before we were seeing the principal
trimmed down. You have to keep your eye on the goal, especially in
the beginning when departments who have never worked together
before (and have, in the past, even been competitive) are joining
forces to address a common issue. So many times we don't really
know what other departments do. You can't give up after one or two
chaotic team meetings that didn't seem to be productive. There's a
light at the end of the tunnel if you are determined to be flexible
and work together as a team to improve patient care. Staff, after all,
are really our most important resource."

Says Bonnie Fossett of her experience with the integration of
QA and CQI: "We are six years into what is often referred to in the
literature as a five-to-ten-year transition. Although I initially
thought that this was far too long, I have come to understand that
the transition is probably never 'complete,' but forever evolving into

a better state of knowledge about process and performance" (Berman, 1995, p. 147).

CQI, as a continual effort to deliver healthcare that meets or exceeds customer expectations, represents a promising approach for improving quality of care while controlling costs (Shortell, Levin, O'Brien, & Hughes, 1995). Yet one of the basic principles of teaching anything new to adults is to help them see that the information is necessary. Mention the word "quality" and visions of clipboards, check-off sheets, and red pens still dance in employees' heads. "All this CQI stuff is getting rid of jobs," groused one nursing assistant. "I can see the handwriting on the wall." When done correctly, however, CQI is a wise investment at the employee, customer, and organizational levels, as it encompasses the timeless maxim of valuing people. The challenge will be the implementation of CQI in an era of budget cutting and increasing change, confusion, and insecurity for American healthcare workers, leaving many feeling inadequate and overwhelmed.

CQI AND THE COMPETITIVE EDGE

When it comes to quality, what you don't know about your customers *can* hurt you. CQI is customer-driven—an absolute obsession with satisfying customers. Through the use of cross-functional, interdisciplinary teams which are fruitful due to the concerted efforts and expertise of many individuals, CQI can bring lasting success to your organization. Managing the future means continually looking at ways to improve quality. And because more effective organizations are also cost effective, CQI saves money and adds to an organization's competitive edge (Koska, 1990). For the real threat in today's changing world of healthcare is not outside competition, but rather internal inefficiency and lack of attention to quality and customers' needs. There is simply no substitute for quality.

Yet we make the idea of CQI far more complicated than it needs to be. While CQI takes time to fully implement, it's one of the most practical approaches to healthcare to ever come down the pike. "It makes sense and that's scary," comments one nursing instructor. CQI removes the "them versus us" barrier of titles, so prevalent in healthcare, and gets departments moving from a "me, mine, and I" frame of reference to one of "we, us, and ours." That's important because, as Crosby (1992) predicts, in the 21st century information will flow up the organization, not down.

Quality and Your Nursing Unit

In most larger healthcare facilities today, there is a quality improvement department (usually accountable to top management) that oversees such functions as CQI, Risk Management, Infection Control, and Utilization Review. Quality improvement staff are also typically involved in employee education about quality issues and the CQI process, and may serve as facilitators for CQI teams. Organizations commonly designate a registered nurse to coordinate and interface nursing quality improvement activities with other departments in the organization. However, with the implementation of CQI and an ever-increasing focus on collaborative efforts, such positions are still evolving.

Some nursing units assign a registered nurse (as a collateral duty) to work in concert with the nurse manager to develop and coordinate unit quality improvement and related staff development activities. Staff education is a definite key to success as CQI represents an entire organizational cultural change. "People don't always understand CQI and that's a major reason why they don't volunteer to participate, especially with teams that involve other departments," observes a quality manager. All staff should be targeted for CQI training, where they are given an opportunity away from their jobs to try on the concept for size.

Whatever the organization's approach to the quality movement, it's always crucial to provide staff with positive feedback. "No one 'oohs and aahs' over things like preventing pressure ulcers," observes a night shift nurse. For a program to be effective, the desired behaviors must be rewarded.

So often we compare ourselves to others and are lulled into thinking the grass is greener on the other side; if there were just enough money and staff, we'd solve our quality problems; if we could just afford the latest cardiac monitors, we'd give better care. It's best in the beginning to embark on a well-defined quality improvement project that will likely reward you with a good return on your investment. As Fran, a nurse on a short-stay unit, recalls: "We got into a wild, hairy project we couldn't possibly maintain, much less move ahead with, given our resources. It reminded me of the time I bought a dress on sale for $30.00, and every time I had it dry-cleaned it cost me $27.00 to have the pleats pressed."

The first step in designing a CQI effort on your nursing unit is to closely examine your key processes and how they affect both quality of care and customer satisfaction. If you hear several nurses in your satellite clinic remark that patients have been complaining about the lack of wheelchair ramps and handicap parking, for example, you may well have a quality issue in regard to access to care. Central to any CQI effort is the question: will this take us from our mission to our vision?

And keep the paperwork in CQI activities to an absolute minimum. While pertinent documentation is essential, nothing is more counterproductive than a quality initiative that appears to be only a "paper shuffle"—a ritual without reason. Organizations should collect data and evaluate improvement on an ongoing basis and in a consistent manner. Data should demonstrate whether changes in functions, processes, and outcomes resulted in measurable improvement; such data is invaluable, concrete feedback for staff. Ask yourself, "Are we duplicating data generated elsewhere? Are our forms unnecessarily complicated?" You're not married to your forms; make them work for you. The JCAHO gives us the flexibility to meet the intent of their standards in a way that best suits our individual settings.

Monitoring and evaluation is to quality care and customer satisfaction what the Good Housekeeping Seal of Approval is to products. Think for a moment to the last time you purchased inferior merchandise or workmanship. Maybe it was Christmas Eve, and when you went to assemble your child's new toy, a part was broken. Remember how disappointed you felt? There was that piece of paper that read, "Inspected by No. 406," but what difference did it make that someone inspected it? That still didn't make it right.

As Marcel Proust observed: "The real voyage of discovery consists not in seeking new landscapes, but in having new eyes." Most people come to work wanting to do a credible job. When staff participate they have a greater interest and investment in CQI. Explore your unit's hidden assets. The key to success in any CQI program is people. Some institutions have adopted a slogan, "QUALITY Begins With 'U'" or "QUALITY Can't Happen Without 'U'" to emphasize that point.

A quality focus helps a department concentrate on the things which really matter—real patient-centered issues, not the trivial pursuit we often find ourselves involved in. "The main thing is to keep the main thing the main thing, and that comes down to patients," as one vice president of nursing is fond of saying.

Take a close look at what you're already doing. So often we feel tugged at every turn, with little patches of QI everywhere. Where is there room for improvement? Solicit the input of all staff, particularly those providing hands-on care. The further away we get from suffering, the more idealistic we tend to become. Frontline caregivers have the inside track on quality, and discounting their input shatters confidence like a delicate china cup broken into a hundred pieces. Brainstorm ideas during unit staff meetings. None of us is as smart as all of us.

It's always preferable to do one or two things really well than to look into a lot of problems and not improve anything. We're a generation who wants things now and every problem solved at once. "It's like trying to take on world hunger instead of taking a bag of groceries to the local food bank," says a unit manager. "It can't be done. Start small and don't make things too complicated. The CQI process takes time, but it's one of the best things to happen to nursing and healthcare."

Share Information

It's important for employees to understand that the quality movement is not just some whizbang new idea dictated from an ivory tower. Many staff continue to see CQI as simply collecting data which sometimes identifies them as the source of the problem, and they can't see the ultimate benefit to the patient.

Post CQI results to show progress and to demonstrate that CQI is far more than plowing through piles of paperwork. "Healthcare is developing a paranoia all its own with all the changes," observes a staff nurse. Invest in building trust, the basis for any CQI program.

When Ford Motor Company was staging its well-remembered comeback, plant managers discussed sensitive financial and quality data with union leaders to break down the "us versus them" barrier. "Opening the books showed the union leaders that we wanted workers to be involved in the company's future, and it let them know precisely where we stood," write Peterson and Hillkirk (1991. p. 28). "Believe me, it was often a very sobering experience. Through the union leaders, we were telling our employees how the world really was. If they, as American workers, weren't willing to fight to improve the company, we could not compete effectively."

That's what CQI is all about. Getting away from hierarchies and into a more collaborative atmosphere where employees are coached and mentored, not scolded—where non-traditional staff who color outside the lines are given a second, longer look.

Accountability for Quality

"We've grown so accustomed to shoddy merchandise and inferior service that we're no longer shocked or offended by them," says a middle-aged man. That point was really brought home when a florist delivered a bouquet of "get well" flowers to my home. As he handed the droopy daises to me, he said, "Hurry and water them. These things are thirsty." The flowers looked worse than I did, but it was his comment that really got me to thinking: How often do we deliver nursing care apologetically? ("I would have done better, but we had two call-ins today.")

A CQI focus, in any industry, means doing the right thing, doing it right the first time, striving for continuous improvement, and satisfying customers. CQI increases individual responsibility by building quality into every step of healthcare and personal accountability into every customer encounter. How an individual measures up to an organization's philosophy of CQI should be a part of the performance appraisal—not merely evaluating their clinical competence, but how they satisfy customers as well.

An Effective Problem Solving Approach

CQI is a highly flexible process that can improve the quality and cost-effectiveness of the complex and changing arena of healthcare and customer satisfaction. Yet if you don't take the time to ascertain the real issue, you may solve the wrong problem or, worse yet, create a new one. This further frustrates staff and customers. Consider developing a flowchart to outline each step in a particular process to more carefully articulate where your system is breaking down. Or you may want to use a "fishbone" cause and effect diagram to evaluate potential causes for identified problems. There are many references which will help you master the numerous tools used in the CQI process to analyze data. To arrive at the right answers, you have to ask the right questions.

We need to examine both unanswered questions and unquestioned answers. Remember, CQI is data driven; quality improvement in healthcare can no longer survive as a soft science and satisfy internal and external customers. Is it really more efficient, and does it contribute to better patient satisfaction, to do all baths on the day tour of duty? As simple as this sounds, have you ever asked your customers for input? All problems may not be readily apparent. If you don't address customer concerns, chances are your competitor will.

We have a tendency in healthcare and in life to solve the wrong problems. This is a waste of valuable time and resources. The people doing the work know best how to solve problems because they know their customers better than anyone.

Let your imagination have free reign. Microsoft says their only factory asset is the human imagination (Peters, 1994). That idea sounds amazingly similar to Einstein's contention that "imagination is more important than knowledge."

Quality and the Future

Through the years, many individuals have attempted to articulate the unique focus of nursing. Over a century ago Florence Nightingale said: "It has been said and written scores of times that every woman makes a good nurse. I believe on the contrary, that the very elements of nursing are all but unknown." While some aspects of nursing elude expression, one facet is crystal clear and transcends the passage of time: Today and in the future, the success of nursing will depend on quality and having a customer-centered focus.

References

Bader, M. M. (1988). Nursing care behaviors that predict patient satisfaction. *Journal of Nursing Quality Assurance, 2*(3), 11-17.

Berglund, R. (1994, March 16). *TQI: Making it happen.* Presented at Managing for Change: Total Quality Improvement Leadership Program, Department of Veterans Affairs, Houston, TX.

Berman, S. (1995). Ending the QA/CQI confusion: An interview with Bonnie Fossett. *Journal of Quality Improvement, 21*(3), 144-147.

Berwick, D. M., Blanton, G. A., & Roessner, J. (1990). *Curing health care: New strategies for quality improvement.* San Francisco: Jossey-Bass, Inc.

Bowers, M. R., Swan, J. E., & Koehler, W. F. (1994). What attributes determine quality and satisfaction with health care delivery? *Health Care Management Review, 19*(4), 49-55.

Brown, S. W., Nelson, A., & Bronkesh, S. J., & Wood, S. D. (1993). *Patient satisfaction pays: Quality service for practice success.* Gaithersburg, MD: Aspen Publishers, Inc.

Cannie, J. K., & Caplin, D. (1991). *Keeping customers for life.* New York: AMACOM.

CHAP. (1995). Informational brochure. New York: Community Health Accreditation Program, Inc.

Codman, E. A. (1916). *A study in hospital efficiency: The first five years.* Boston: Thomas Todd Company.

Crosby, P. B. (1992). *Completeness: Quality for the 21st century.* New York: Penguin Books USA, Inc.

Deming, W. E. (1986). *Out of the crisis.* Cambridge, MA: Massachusetts Institute of Technology Center for Advanced Engineering Study.

Ente, B. H. (1994). Joint Commission to release organization-specific performance information. *Joint Commission Perspectives, 14*(5), 1, 6-7.

George, S., & Weimerskirch, A. (1994). *Total quality management: Strategies and techniques proven at today's most successful companies.* New York: John Wiley and Sons, Inc.

Greene, J. (1995, May 29). System hospitals earn high JCAHO marks. *Modern Healthcare,* 33-34.

Haddock, C. C., Nosky, C., Fargason, C. A., & Kurz, R. S. (1995). The impact of CQI on human resources management. *Hospitals and Health Services Administration, 40*(1), 138-153.

Hall, J. A., Roter, D. L., & Katz, N. R. (1988). Task versus socioemotional behaviors in patients. *Medical Care, 25,* 399-412.

JCAHO. (1994). *The Joint Commission 1995 comprehensive accreditation manual for hospitals. Volume I: Standards.* Oakbrook Terrace, IL: Author.

Joint Commission on Accreditation of Healthcare Organizations. (1990). *Primer on indicator development and application: Measuring quality in healthcare.* Oakbrook Terrace, IL: Author.

Joint Commission. (1994). *Joint Commission Perspectives, 14*(2), 1-9.

Koska, M. T. (1989, Feb. 5). Quality—Thy name is nursing care, CEOs say. *Hospitals, 32.*

Koska, M. T. (1990, March 5). High-quality care and hospital projects: Is there a link? *Hospitals,* 62-63.

Merriam Webster, Inc. (1991). *Webster's ninth new collegiate dictionary.* Springfield, MA: Author.

Moore, N., & Moore, K. (1993). *Patient-focused healing.* San Francisco: Jossey-Bass Publishers.

Omachonu, V. K. (1990). Quality of care and the patient: New criteria for evaluation. *Health Care Management Review, 15*(4), 40-50.

Peters, T. (1994). *The Tom Peters seminar: Crazy times call for crazy organizations.* New York: Vintage Books.

Peterson, D. E., & Hillkirk, J. (1991). *A better idea: Redefining the way Americans work.* Boston: Houghton Mifflin Co.

Shortell, S. M. (1995, June). The future of hospitals and health care management. *FORUM: VA Health Services Research and Development,* 1-3.

Shortell, S. M., Levin, D. Z., O'Brien, J. L., & Hughes, F. X. (1995). Assessing the evidence on CQI: Is the glass half empty or half full? *Hospital and Health Services Administration, 40*(1), 4-24.

Staff. (1993, February 5). Putting patients first: Hospitals work to define patient-centered care. *Hospitals,* 14-26.

The National Association of Quality Assurance Professionals. (1991). *Guide to healthcare quality management.* Deerfield, IL: Author.

Tucker, R. B. (1991). *Managing the future.* New York: G.P. Putnam's Sons.

Turner, J. T., & Matthews, K. A. (1991, Summer). Measuring adolescent satisfaction with nursing care in an ambulatory setting. *The ABNF Journal,* 48-52.

Whiteley, R. C. (1991). *The customer driven company: Moving from talk to action.* Reading, MA: Addison-Wesley Publishing Co.

Ziegenfuss, J. T., & O'Rourke, P. (1995). Ombudsmen, patient complaints, and total quality management. *Journal of Quality Improvement, 21*(3), 133-142.

Chapter 4

YES, PATIENTS DO HAVE RIGHTS

What we really need is state-of-the-art technology combined with
state-of-the-heart staff.
— Roberta Messner

Protecting and preserving the rights of patients is an important part of patient satisfaction because, when such rights are violated, it's as if one's personal self is diminished. In her article, "Meeting Consumer Expectations," Roxane Spitzer (1988) cites a number of such customer complaints (gleaned from several studies) that point to important patient rights issues:

- Nurses were uninvolved and dehumanizing.

- Nurses distanced themselves and avoided interaction.

- Staff did not involve the patient[s] in decision making.

- Nurses focused on the equipment and procedure rather than on the patient[s].

- Nurses showed lack of empathy or openness to patients' feelings.

- Nurses and physicians, in the patients' presence, discussed their cases in the third person with another professional. (pp. 32-33)

All clinical care and research should be provided with respect for the patient's dignity as a unique human being with fundamental human, civil, constitutional, and statutory rights. According to the JCAHO (1994), healthcare organizations should respect patient rights and personal dignity, and provide considerate, respectful care based on individual needs. This includes affirming the patients' right to make decisions affecting care and assisting them to exercise those rights while accepting responsibility for personal decisions.

The American Hospital Association (1992) has published a Patient's Bill of Rights based on a foundation of respect for human beings as individuals and emphasizing active patient participation (Figure 4.1).

FIGURE 4.1 A PATIENT'S BILL OF RIGHTS
Patient and Community Relations

INTRODUCTION

Effective health care requires collaboration between patients and physicians and other health care professionals. Open and honest communication, respect for personal and professional values, and sensitivity to differences are integral to optimal patient care. As the setting for the provision of health services, hospitals must provide a foundation for understanding and respecting the rights and responsibilities of patients, their families, physicians, and other caregivers. Hospitals must ensure a health care ethic that respects the role of patients in decision making about treatment choices and other aspects of their care. Hospitals must be sensitive to cultural, racial, linguistic, religious, age, gender, and other differences as well as the needs of persons with disabilities.

The American Hospital Association presents A Patient's Bill of Rights with the expectation that it will contribute to more effective patient care and be supported by the hospital on behalf of the institution, its medical staff, employees, and patients. The American Hospital Association encourages health care institutions to tailor this bill of rights to their patient community by translating and/or simplifying the language of this bill of rights as may be necessary to ensure that patients and their families understand their rights and responsibilities.

BILL OF RIGHTS

1. The patient has the right to considerate and respectful care.

2. The patient has the right to and is encouraged to obtain from physicians and other direct caregivers relevant, current, and understandable information concerning diagnosis, treatment, and prognosis.

   Except in emergencies when the patient lacks decision-making capacity and the need for treatment is urgent, the patient is entitled to the opportunity to discuss and request information related to the specific procedures and/or treatments, the risks involved, the possible length of recuperation, and the medically reasonable alternatives and their accompanying risks and benefits.

   Patients have the right to know the identity of physicians, nurses, and others involved in their care, as well as when those involved are students, residents, or other trainees. The patient also has the right to know the immediate and long-term financial implications of treatment choices, insofar as they are known.

3. The patient has the right to make decisions about the plan of care prior to and during the course of treatment and to refuse a recommended treatment or plan of care to the extent permitted by law and hospital policy and to be informed of the medical consequences of this action. In case of such refusal, the patient is entitled to other appropriate care and services that the hospital provides or transfer to another hospital. The hospital should notify patients of any policy that might affect patient choice within the institution.

4. The patient has the right to have an advance directive (such as a living will, health care proxy, or durable power of attorney for health care) concerning treatment or designating a surrogate decision maker with the expectation that the hospital will honor the intent of that directive to the extent permitted by law and hospital policy.

   Health care institutions must advise patients of their rights under state law and hospital policy to make informed medical choices, ask if the patient has an advance directive, and include that information in patient records. The patient has the right to timely information about hospital policy that may limit its ability to implement fully a legally valid advance directive.

   The patient has the right to every consideration of privacy. Case discussion, consultation, examination, and treatment should be conducted so as to protect each patient's privacy.

6. The patient has the right to expect that all communications and records pertaining to his/her care will be treated as confidential by the hospital, except in cases such as suspected abuse and public health hazards when reporting is permitted or required by law. The patient has the right to expect that the hospital will emphasize the confidentiality of this information when it releases it to any other parties entitled to review information in these records.

7. The patient has the right to review the records pertaining to his/her medical care and to have the information explained or interpreted as necessary, except when restricted by law.

8. The patient has the right to expect that, within its capacity and policies, a hospital will make reasonable response to the request of a patient for appropriate and medically indicated care and services. The hospital must provide evaluation, service, and/or referral as indicated by the urgency of the case. When medically appropriate and legally permissible, or when a patient has so requested, a patient may be transferred to another facility. The institution to which the patient is to be transferred must first have accepted the patient for transfer. The patient must also have the benefit of complete information and explanation concerning the need for, risks, benefits, and alternatives to such a transfer.

9. The patient has the right to ask and be informed of the existence of business relationships among the hospital, educational institutions, other health care providers, or payers that may influence the patient's treatment and care.

10. The patient has the right to consent to or decline to participate in proposed research studies or human experimentation affecting care and treatment or requiring direct patient involvement, and to have those studies fully explained prior to consent. A patient who declines to participate in research or experimentation is entitled to the most effective care that the hospital can otherwise provide.

11. The patient has the right to expect reasonable continuity of care when appropriate and to be informed by physicians and other caregivers of available and realistic patient care options when hospital care is no longer appropriate.

12. The patient has the right to be informed of hospital policies and practices that relate to patient care, treatment, and responsibilities. The patient has the right to be informed of available resources for resolving disputes, grievances, and conflicts, such as ethics committees, patient representatives, or other mechanisms available in the institution. The patient has the right to be informed of the hospital's charges for services and available payment methods.

    The collaborative nature of health care requires that patients, or their families/surrogates, participate in their care. The effectiveness of care and patient satisfaction with the course of treatment depend, in part, on the patient fulfilling certain responsibilities. Patients are responsible for providing information about past illnesses, hospitalizations, medications, and other matters related to health status. To participate effectively in decision making, patients must be encouraged to take responsibility for requesting additional information or clarification about their health status or treatment when they do not fully understand information and instructions. Patients are also responsible for ensuring that the health care institution has a copy of their written advance directive if they have one. Patients are responsible for informing their physicians and other caregivers if they anticipate problems in following prescribed treatment.

Patients should also be aware of the hospital's obligation to be reasonably efficient and equitable in providing care to other patients and the community. The hospital's rules and regulations are designed to help the hospital meet this obligation. Patients and their families are responsible for making reasonable accommodations to the needs of the hospital, other patients, medical staff, and hospital employees. Patients are responsible for providing necessary information for insurance claims and for working with the hospital to make payment arrangements, when necessary.

A person's health depends on much more than health care services. Patients are responsible for recognizing the impact of their lifestyle on their personal health.

CONCLUSION

Hospitals have many functions to perform, including the enhancement of health status, health promotion, and the prevention and treatment of injury and disease; the immediate and ongoing care and rehabilitation of patients; the education of health professionals, patients, and the community; and research. All these activities must be conducted with an overriding concern for the values and dignity of patients.

(Reprinted with permission from the American Hospital Association ©1992)

Many organizations include these expectations (adapted to their specific patient population) in handbooks which should be available to all patients on orientation to the agency or admission to the hospital (Figure 4.2).

FIGURE 4.2 Patient Rights and Responsibilities

At Cabell Huntington Hospital, we are committed to giving the best care to you without regard to your race, color, religion, national origin or source of payment, and without regard to disability. You should become an active participant in your health care process. To do this, it is important that you understand your rights and responsibilities.

Your Rights

1. You have the right to obtain from your physician information necessary to give informed consent prior to the start of any procedure or treatment.
2. You have the right to receive general information about hospital rules and regulations and the name of anyone providing you with services and his or her relationship to the hospital.
3. You have the right to be well informed about your illness, possible treatments, likely outcomes, and to discuss this information with your doctor.
4. You have the right to a living will, or medical power of attorney to express your choices about your future care if you cannot speak for yourself.
5. You have the right to privacy. We will respect your privacy as it relates to you and your medical care program.
6. You have the right to receive information about charges billed to your account.

Your Responsibility

1. It is your responsibility to provide us with information about your health, past illness, hospital stays, and medicine.
2. It is your responsibility to follow instructions given by your physician and staff and ask questions when you do not understand.
3. It is your responsibility to be considerate of the needs of other patients, and follow guidelines concerning smoking, visitors, noise and conduct.
4. It is your responsibility to provide information to the hospital about your ability to pay for services.

For additional information regarding your rights and responsibilities as a patient, please request a copy of the hospital policy on Patient Rights and Responsibilities from your nurse or the Patient Representative.

All of us at Cabell Huntington Hospital want the best care for our patients and we want your stay to be as comfortable as possible. If you have any concerns over services provided and if there is any way we can serve you better, please contact the Patient Representative.

(Reprinted with permission from Cabell Huntington Hospital, Huntington, West Virginia)

What Do Patients Have to Say?

In a large study involving 225 hospitals in 32 states (139,830 patient surveys), 15 top indicators of overall patient satisfaction were identified. While all of these attributes may not apply to your organization, notice how many have to do with basic rights as well as the quality of communication:

1. Staff concern for your privacy

2. Staff sensitivity to inconvenience of sickness and hospitalization

3. Adequacy of information given to family about your condition and treatment

4. Overall cheerfulness of hospital

5. Nurses' attitude to your calling them

6. Extent to which nurses took your problem seriously

7. Nurses' attention to your personal and special needs

8. Courtesy of technician who took your blood

9. Technicians' explanations of tests and treatments

10. Likelihood of recommending hospital

11. Nurses' friendliness

12. Nurses' promptness in responding to call button

13. Nurses' information about tests and treatments

14. Technical skill of the nurses

15. Skill of technician who took your blood[*]

---

*Copyright 1992, Press, Ganey Associates. Used with permission

Notice that privacy was the number one concern. Interestingly, patients cared for in larger hospitals express more dissatisfaction in regard to privacy than those cared for in smaller hospitals (Press, Ganey Associates, 1992, p. 17).

"When my 32-year-old brother was flat on his back with a crushed vertebrae," remembers Jenna, "a nurse stood in the hallway and yelled, 'Mr. Sampson, do you need a urinal? Do you need to pee?' He was mortified. It didn't matter that he had an excellent neurosurgeon and orthopedist, and received wonderful nursing care. Even today, the fact that a nurse did that to him causes him more distress than the physical chronic back pain he continues to experience."

"I believe patients should feel like they're the most important thing you've got to do all day," says a staff nurse. "I've found if you approach nursing in an ethical manner, you will always provide quality care. Whenever you find yourself strapped for time or in a dilemma, always ask, 'What is best for the patient?'"

ACCESS TO CARE

Access to healthcare is an increasingly serious problem in America, and is of concern to nurses. Margie, a community health nurse, contends, "No one in a country as affluent as ours should have to go without healthcare. It just doesn't make sense."

Access to care incorporates five core components: "availability, accessibility, accommodation, affordability, and acceptability" (Schiff, Goldberg, & Ansell, 1992, p. 139). Each year one million American families are denied medical care because of financial reasons (Woolhandler & Himmelstein, 1989). Groups who have difficulty with accessibility include those in rural areas, the indigent, undocumented workers, minorities, the mentally handicapped, children, and young adults (Schiff et al., 1992).

WALK A MILE IN MY SHOES

"If you want to know what it's like to be a patient, be a patient," says Nona, a nurse who has endured nine surgical procedures in the past 4 years due to injuries sustained in an auto accident. But as Johnson and Wilson (1984, p. 37) point out, "Before I can walk in another person's shoes, I must first take off my own." Observes a respiratory therapist: "Sometimes that means we healthcare workers must remove the professional masks we often hide behind. It's like someone once said, 'A mask tells you more than a face.'" So much of what we do distances us from our patients; gloves, goggles, and other protective gear, for example, as well as the explosion of technology in modern healthcare.

The late Norman Cousins, in a commencement address to the George Washington University Medical School, made some wonderful observations about the physician's critical role in communication. He said that patients come to their doctor with not one, but two diseases—the actual physical problem and panic.

"I pray that when he goes into a patient's room," Cousins said, "the physician will recognize that the main distance is not from the door to the bed but from the patient's eyes to his own, and the shortest distance between those two points is a horizontal straight line—the kind of straight line that works best when the physician bends low to the patient's loneliness, fear, and pain, and the overwhelming sense of mortality that comes flooding up out of the unknown, and when the physician's hand on the patient's shoulder or arm is a shelter against darkness" (Gerteis, Edgman-Levitan, Daley, & Delbanco, 1993, p. 78).

A patient's call light buzzes just as you're preparing to pass medications . . . a dying patient's wife requests to speak with you five minutes before your shift ends. "Sometimes a patient will stop me in the middle of something and ask me to get them a blanket or a sip of water," says Donna. "In the big scheme of everything nurses do, it doesn't seem like much. But I've realized so many times, a patient asks for something small when they are afraid of something big. And if I can make them feel comforted for one moment, I've accomplished something."

JUST WHAT DO PATIENTS WANT?

Patients clearly desire considerate, respectful care geared toward their individual needs. Keep in mind that a basic tenet of nursing is patient-centered practice. As healthcare clinicians we should support patients' rights to make decisions about their care, including the decision to stop treatment, to the extent permitted by law (JCAHO, 1994).

"One of the most important roles a nurse can play is to help patients and families clarify their wishes," contends Sue, a nurse on a geriatrics unit. "Be attuned to people and you'll know when the right moment has arrived. When you're administering a tube feeding to a terminally ill woman and her husband asks, 'What are you trying to do, get her ready to enter a marathon?' you have the perfect opening to discuss what they expect and want. And when the patient admitted in respiratory distress tells you, 'I don't want any artificial hookups,' that's a cue to ensure that advance directives are adequately discussed with her."

"One of the most memorable moments in my nursing career," recalls a former ICU nurse, "occurred early in the AIDS epidemic. I was caring for a young attorney in the end stage of the disease when a lab tech came into his room to draw arterial blood gases. The attorney's eyes darted all over the room like he was afraid someone was going to pounce on him, and I'll never forget what he said: 'NO! NO! The patient has the right to refuse treatment!' He died later that day, but there was such authority and dignity in those last words."

INFORMED CHOICE

Patients (and designated family members) are entitled to a clear, concise explanation of their condition and any proposed treatments or procedures, including the potential benefits and complications, so they can truly give informed consent.

"When I was having surgery, a team of doctors thundered into my room, shoved a piece of paper under my nose, and said, 'Sign this,'" remembers a construction worker. "I was trying to read it when one of them said, 'If you can't read, just make an X.' I made a big joke out of it and said, 'I can't do that. That's my dad's name.' But all kidding aside, I knew my rights. I wasn't about to put my name on something I didn't understand."

It's important that customers know what to expect as well. In interviewing patients who had undergone bypass surgery at one group of hospitals, the most common complaint was that no one explained they would wake up on a ventilator. Patients have the right to information, including alternative treatment measures, and such information leads to better outcomes, such as decreased anxiety and pain (Koska, 1992).

"When I looked up that new drug I'm taking," says Nancy, who has been having TIAs, "I learned the side effects are male-pattern hair loss, a deepening of my voice, and hair on my face. Why didn't someone tell me I was going to look like a wrestler? I think I'd just as soon have a stroke."

And don't forget family members. As the distraught husband of an I.C.U. patient remarked to another visitor in the family waiting area: "They told me my wife's condition hadn't changed, but they never really told me what her condition was. I don't know how to plan for anything."

"No one seemed to talk directly to me," writes Ivy Bailey, RN (1985, p. 53), who underwent open heart surgery. Pressure on her optic nerve limited her vision and made her feel as if she were seeing the world through a peephole. She remembers a nurse who came into her room, whisked off the blankets, turned her over, and took a rectal temperature—all without uttering a word to her. She concluded that what nurses say to patients may be just as important as what they do for them.

THE RIGHT TO REFUSE TREATMENT

On admission to the hospital patients should be informed of their right to accept or refuse treatment, give advance directives regarding the use of life-supporting treatment, and appoint someone to make medical decisions should they become unable to make sound decisions. Documents such as the Living Will and Durable

Power of Attorney for healthcare offer assurance that their wishes are known and can be carried out whenever legally possible. When 68-year-old Joseph Yang had surgery to correct an aortic aneurysm, for example, he told his family and his physician that he did not want to have extensive life support measures should major complications occur. He also gave his oldest son power of attorney to make decisions for him should Mr. Yang become unable to do so.

Many states have made statutory provisions for both types of advance directive documents: the healthcare Power of Attorney (or healthcare proxy) and the Living Will (sometimes called natural death declarations). The patient then indicates treatment preferences (often about life-sustaining care) and/or designates a surrogate decision-maker in the event he or she no longer can make decisions.

JCAHO surveyors evaluate if advance directives are documented in the patient's medical record. They also scrutinize charts to see if advance directives are reconsidered when patients are transferred to or from intensive care units.

"It was such a relief when the nurse brought up the subject of whether I even wanted to be put back on the respirator again," remembers Mary, a patient with end-stage emphysema who had previously spent six months on a ventilator. "It had been wearing me and my family down, but no one would dare utter the words. My daughter later laughed that she was afraid people would think she was after my money if she ever suggested discontinuing the respirator."

"I find a lot of patients don't understand what an advance directive really is," says a pulmonologist. "I'll often ask them, 'Have you ever put anything in writing about medical decisions to be made if for some reason you weren't able to make them for yourself?'"

THE EFFECT OF ILLNESS ON THE PATIENT

Ethicist David Roy cites a number of consequences that serious illness may have on a person. It interrupts their sense of independence and control, giving power to others, often strangers; alters their view of the world, and the world's view of them; and changes the very fabric of relationships (Mount, 1993). Major illness affects the biological, mental, social, and spiritual dimensions of life. Roles and relationships are altered, physical ability and body functioning impaired, lifelong beliefs challenged, and personal identity threatened.

Bernie Siegel, M.D., once humorously recommended that patients be given a water gun on admission to the hospital and told that they have permission to use it when someone violates their boundaries—a way of maintaining control in an out-of-control environment. It's sometimes difficult for healthcare workers to fully appreciate how out of control patients feel when they leave their secure, familiar world for the often frightening, dehumanizing land of the medical unknown.

A LITTLE RESPECT, PLEASE

When it comes to matters of patient satisfaction, respect and common courtesy may be the major area where things go wrong, say authors Tanenbaum and Berman (1993). Respect is important in any relationship, but is never more critical, from both a therapeutic and a risk management perspective, than in the depersonalized healthcare environment. The fundamental, guiding principle and "golden rule of thumb" in caring for patients is respect, (Applegate, 1993, p. 61). This concept is emphasized in the ANA Code for Nurses with Interpretive Statements as the "supreme moral principle" from which all others flow (Applegate, 1993, p. 61).

"Book sense and horse sense are far from the same thing," quips an assembly line worker from Detroit. Yet patients are all-too-often judged by their level of education and their titles, instead of being approached as individuals worthy of respect. "The only way them medical people measure worth is by how many years you went to school and how much stuff you've got," adds another patient. "If you're poor and don't have much schoolin', your opinion ain't worth nothin'."

Patients who don't feel respected are more likely to sue their caregivers, and lack of respect further compounds the loss of control a patient is experiencing as a result of being dependent. But

more than that, respect is at the core of every relationship. It causes marriages and friendships to crumble, and is a major problem
in patients' perceptions of healthcare. "Some of these doctors talk
at you, not *to* you," complains a patient with hepatitis. "The one
they assigned to my case never even introduced himself. I find him
disrespectful, even though they tell me he's supposed to be a pretty good doctor. I like for people to get on my level."

Acceptance of an individual's values and beliefs communicates
respect for the whole person, especially as we move toward a more
global, culturally diverse society. A nurse who works in the ER of a
small hospital serving Native Americans explains, "It's not uncommon for medicine men to accompany a patient and family when
someone is very ill, and we always allow them to perform their traditional rituals in addition to our use of modern medical treatment.
And you know what? It makes an astonishing positive difference
in the patient's overall recovery."

Perceived lack of respect takes many forms. "When I was in the
hospital," observes another patient recalling a well-remembered
scene, "there were 15-20 doctors tripping through my room every
morning, and not a one of them would tell me what was going on."
Echoes another dissatisfied patient: "All they do at my HMO is say,
'Yep, yep, yep.' They don't want to know how I feel. They want to tell
me how I ought to feel. I'm a person, too, and no one's paying attention to that. I want to scream, 'May I say something?'"

A patient who lives in rural Appalachia once told me about a
couple of new doctors they'd hired at his clinic. "They really take
time to get to know you," he said, "and so they're real popular with
all the patients. I mentioned it to one of the docs who had been
working there a long time. 'Oh, they had to find a few doctors who
could say "Ain't,"' he hooted. But I think there was more to it than
them hiring a bunch of good ol' boys.'"

Staying true to your word is another way of showing customers
respect. "One of the most frustrating aspects of the medical profession is their seeming disregard for following through on promises,"
observes a nursing home administrator. "Patients and family members take this very seriously, especially older people who were
taught that a person's word was the window to their character."

Make it a policy to be dependable and consistent in your approach to customers, and don't make promises you may not be able to keep. This is the very foundation of building trust in the nurse-patient relationship (Messner & Ward, 1989). It's far better to say "I'll try my best to get to that this morning" than to assure a patient you'll do something at 10 am, and then renege on that promise.

WOULD YOU DO THE SAME THING IF A LOVED ONE WAS WATCHING?

"I hope if I ever get real ill, someone preserves my dignity," says Janet, whose father recently died in the hospital. "I was raised in an extremely modest home, and here was this nurse taking a rectal temperature in full view of everyone in the hallway. Of course, she didn't know I was there. She didn't even explain what she was doing to him, and she moved him around like a sack of potatoes." The media teaches consumers to be suspicious of healthcare workers and institutions, and for that reason even the most innocent acts can be misconstrued.

"Families have it as hard or harder than the patient," remarks a hospital chaplain. "The patient is often sleeping, medicated, or involved in some way with the treatment team, while the family who loves this person dearly is left to sit and wait. Often no one tells them anything about what is going on, and they are left to their own interpretations of what is happening."

AREN'T ALL PATIENTS THE SAME?

A friend who is studying to be a gerontology nurse practitioner remembers the time her own grandmother was gravely ill in the hospital. Betty has long been fascinated with the unique strengths of elderly people, so she asked the nurse: "Don't you just love working with older patients?" The nurse shot her a quizzical look and replied, "As far as I'm concerned, if you've seen one, you've seen them all." But are they all alike?

While it is true that human beings are similar in more ways than we're different, one of the greatest sources of dissatisfaction among all patients is not being treated as individuals. "I'll tell you what patients really want," says Becky, who wears a shirt announcing, "HAIR BY CHEMO," given to her by the nurses at the cancer center. "It's to be treated special . . . like you're the only one. Cancer is so harsh, and that soft, personal touch really gets you through some tough times."

CAN YOU KEEP A SECRET?

"I told the nurse at the mental health center about a problem I was having with my bills and that busybody blabbed it to everyone," says Tara, a member of Debtors' Anonymous, who is worried about her husband discovering her $30,000 credit card debt. "She promised she wouldn't tell, and now my husband's threatening to divorce me."

If a patient reveals something that must be shared with other caregivers, explain that to them before they tell you. But if not sharing it won't interfere with the quality of their care, or isn't an issue with legal, moral, or ethical implications (such as child or elder abuse or certain infectious diseases), keep it to yourself. Even though much of hospital lore can be quite entertaining to others, resist the urge to tell even your best friend. As a nursing instructor once wisely told her new students: "What you see here, what you hear here, let it stay here." First do no harm.

Look closely at the procedures at your institution which compromise patient confidentiality. "When I was a patient, they posted my weight in big, black letters on a bulletin board in the nurses' station," remembers Alyce, who was hospitalized for congestive heart failure. "All my adult life I'd managed to keep my weight a secret, but no more. They don't even do that at Weight Watchers."

On your OB unit, do you list the number of "abortions" your patients have had on a public bulletin board? To the staff, that term means miscarriages, but to visitors, it may carry an entirely different connotation. How about the sign-in sheet at your office or clinic? Does it ask for information a patient might prefer others in the waiting room wouldn't know? Do you discuss lab results within earshot of other patients? Fax the findings of diagnostic testing to institutions across town? All of these procedures potentially impinge on patient rights.

What about your institution's overhead paging system? A patient tells the story of when he left the clinic waiting area to buy a cup of coffee from the vending machine. "Next thing I knew, the operator was announcing, 'Jim Smith, please return to the Mental Health Clinic,'" he recalls.

"When I had my eye worked on, I'll tell you what impressed me most with the office staff," says an 83-year-old lady. "They held everything in the strictest confidence and gave me total privacy. There weren't any doors leading to other rooms like in some of those places. And they didn't run from room to room talking about other patients or get on the phone and discuss someone's whole medical history right in front of you. I just hate those offices with those paper-thin walls. If I want someone to know my business, I'll tell them myself. I don't need some doctor or nurse to broadcast it."

HONORING CONFIDENTIALITY

The principle of confidentiality requires that nurses respect all privileged information about their patients. Nurses and other caregivers have knowledge of many private and sensitive details. Patients must be able to trust that their confidences will be kept, no matter what.

"We can inadvertently breach confidentiality when we're really trying to show concern," says a nurse employed in a cardiologist's office. "For years I'd ask new patients, 'Do you know so and so?' My rationale was, of course, trying to establish common ground. But experience has taught me that patients are often uncomfortable with that and fear I might divulge their condition to our mutual friends. I've learned to cut the small talk and really hone in on my patients' needs."

Another problem occurs when friends or relatives ask for information about a patient. Such issues should be handled tactfully but firmly. "A lady came up to me at a P.T.A. meeting and inquired about a patient on my unit who was the daughter of a mutual friend," says Nan, a pediatric nurse clinical specialist. "It really put me on the spot for a moment. Then I realized that part of being a patient advocate is protecting the patient's privacy. I affirmed her concern, but explained that she would have to receive that information from the family."

Rural nurses find themselves in particularly precarious situations regarding confidentiality. They may be queried at the grocery store or post office about how a patient's labor is progressing, for example, placing them in an extremely awkward situation (Ethics, 1993). Keep in mind that whenever people experience a loss of control, privacy becomes all the more important. Even something as seemingly insignificant as opening a patient's get-well card can be distressing.

An important issue of confidentiality is to provide a place where the families of critical care and surgical patients can process the news far from the maddening crowd (Long & Greeneich, 1994). Telephones should be in an area where families can discuss the intimate details of life and death decisions without concern that someone is eavesdropping.

A patient has the right to expect confidentiality within reasonable parameters. Technical advances have made sensitive data more available to a host of people, and the right to confidentiality has become a very real concern. It's estimated that as many as 75 people have access to a patient's medical record. A good rule of thumb is that confidentiality is breached unless healthcare workers have a right or a need to know the information, not just because they work in an organization. All persons involved with patient-specific health information must be committed to an ethical code and protective of privacy issues (Milholland, 1994).

With the advent of the computer-based medical record, a patient's entire life history is available, allowing us to network with other healthcare agencies as never before. Yet with this new technology comes responsibility to protect your patients' privacy (Frawley, 1994). Just because patients' incomes are available on the computer, for instance, doesn't give us the right to access that information.

Take care not to release sensitive information by telephone. Follow your hospital's procedure for release of healthcare information. Some hospitals, for example, use a password to ensure that staff are indeed speaking to an authorized family member. Sometimes (such as on psychiatry units) it's a violation of confidentiality to even confirm that a patient is hospitalized on your unit. Any media inquiries should be referred to the appropriate hospital spokesperson.

And by all means, don't talk in public about your patients. "I was dining in a very nice restaurant," recalls a businessman, "and a group of nurses from the community hospital were lunching at the table next to me. One of them remarked, 'I gave that Mr. Hatten the wrong meds this morning, but, you know, with most of our patients it doesn't make any difference.' I listened closely until I found out where they work. I'll certainly think twice before taking my business there." As JCAHO surveyors assess patient care areas, they, too, are ever-astute to confidentiality and privacy issues: if privacy is assured when data are collected, if exam doors are kept closed, and if patient-sensitive information is maintained away from public areas.

DON'T LABEL ME

A single male observed the notation "resides with male" in his chart when his records were photocopied for a disability claim. "The only male I live with is Bob, my cat," he says. "Do they always make such assumptions without asking questions?"

One day I overheard a physician discussing a patient's prescription refills within earshot of an entire office waiting room. "I'm not giving you any more nerve pills," she blared into the phone. After slamming down the receiver she hollered to a colleague, "That Mr. Throckmorton ... I'm sick and tired of his drug-seeking behavior." I couldn't help but wonder, did anyone else besides me know who she was talking about?

Do I Smell Alcohol?

Don't assume a patient has been drinking just because they're staggering, combative, have slurred speech, an unusual odor on their breath, or even have a diagnosis of alcoholism. "One evening when I was working E.R.," remembers Brenda, "the police brought in a woman who was found wandering on the street, and was well-known to us for her drinking problem. She was irritable, argumentative, and vomiting, and appeared to be intoxicated. They placed her in a holding room to be examined by the psychiatrist. Thirty minutes later, a nurse found her unresponsive. The truth was, this time she hadn't been drinking at all. She'd been beaten by her boyfriend and had a head injury."

Is Honesty the Best Policy?

Bill, a psychologist, says there's honesty and there's brutal honesty. It's important to tell the truth, but temper the truth with kindness. When Judy was diagnosed with pancreatic cancer, her doctor told her bluntly she'd be dead in six months. While her prognosis was indeed poor, how much better would the quality of her last days have been had the news been delivered with compassion and a measure of hope. Sometimes healthcare workers are afraid of giving patients false hope. But there's always something to hope for, even in the gravest of circumstances: a friendship can be mended, a family feud resolved.

As clinicians, we often speak curtly out of frustration and our own pain and feelings of inadequacy or powerlessness. But the end of life is not necessarily synonymous with the end of living. A 70-year-old grandmother of 10 who was a home hospice patient comes to mind. "The last three months of my life were the best of all," she said. "I'd always wanted to learn to drive so I could take my grandchildren to school." And despite colon cancer with liver metastasis, she did just that. It's as her hospice nurse observed: "'No Code' doesn't mean 'No Care.' Honesty sets the stage for the most poignant caring of all."

"When you're feeling like there's nothing else you can do for a patient," reminds a psychiatric nurse, "keep in mind, the most important resource for nursing is interacting with them honestly, heart to heart" (Lewis & Morton, 1994). That's how caring, understanding, and compassion ultimately touch a patient. Sometimes our most therapeutic moments are when we have no idea of how therapeutic we really are.

Nurses need to remain aware of the importance of the physician-patient relationship and its impact on the nursing role, especially in the realm of giving information. It is the physician's responsibility to inform the patient about medical issues, not the nurse's. In some cases a patient may choose not to know the truth. All caregivers should be sensitive to the patient's wishes and the need to maintain the caregiver-patient relationship (Applegate, 1993).

There are more words in the English language than in any other tongue, and that translates into innumerable opportunities for misinterpretation. Remember in grade school when kids would chant, "Sticks and stones may break my bones, but words will never hurt me?" That's not so. Words have tremendous power. They can destroy or build up. They can hurt or heal, and honest communication should never be destructive. Language has the power to move and, in some ways, even transform the human heart, says Frederick Buechner (1993). The bottom line is, "How can we better communicate in our organization to better serve and improve the outcomes of our customers?"

WHAT ROLE DOES CULTURE PLAY?

At times, nurses become so caught up in a patient's physiological problems that they neglect to consider the person as a whole, or at best give only superficial credence to the sociocultural, psychological, and spiritual realms. Healing involves "a process of bringing all parts of one's self together at deep levels of inner knowing, leading toward an integration and balance, with each part having equal importance and value" (Dossey & Keegan, 1995, p. 220).

Science and technology alone aren't enough. When interacting with a patient and family of a different culture, take time to learn about their values and beliefs. The stoicism your patient is exhibiting may be cultural in origin. Likewise, the patient who thinks "people come to the hospital to die" may be giving you clues to their cultural heritage (Lipkin & Cohen, 1992). And be sensitive to the impact of culture on a person's illness and treatment, rather than judging and reacting. Take it slowly, to develop a foundation of trust. As Press (1984) says, healthcare is experiencing a crisis of trust which adversely affects patient satisfaction and is partially responsible for the increase in medical malpractice claims.

In some Navajo clans, people aren't permitted to die indoors, explains a nurse who works with this patient population. The dying person is carried outside so when death releases their chindi (ghost), it can lose itself in the vastness of the sky. "In another tribe," continues Larry, a nurse practitioner on an Indian reservation, "during the first year after death, family and loved ones don't emotionally let go, but rather postpone surrendering the soul to the spirit world for a year. They call this ceremony 'the wiping of the tears.'"

Terminology gets tricky, too, when working with different cultures. Sandra, a physician's assistant who moved from upstate New York to rural Kentucky, relates this story: "A gentleman came to my office and told me he 'liked to died.' Of course, I thought that meant he was having suicidal ideation, and I asked for a stat psych consult. Later, the psychiatrist burst into my office laughing, and informed me it was just a figure of speech. The guy had merely been in a lot of discomfort when he took a bowel prep for a barium enema."

Don't discount lay remedies either. "When I moved to North Carolina, one of the locals told me to make a paste of Adolph's meat tenderizer and apply it to my bee sting," recalls a school nurse. "I'd tried everything else, so I figured it couldn't hurt. To my surprise, it actually did relieve the pain and swelling and itching. But it taught me an even more valuable lesson: there's wisdom in 'them thar hills.'"

A Filipino lady relates this story: "My daughter had a stillborn son—our first grandchild—and our whole family was simply devastated. The nurse bathed and dressed the baby in his beautiful blue terry cloth outfit, wrapped him in a soft cuddly blanket, and let us hold him and sing a lullaby. I can still smell his silky, talc-scented skin and remember that kind nurse's loving touch. It helped us know this child as a real little person, and begin our mourning."

Some hospitals have instituted a protocol to help families deal with the loss of stillborn and terminally ill infants that includes taking a photograph of the infant for the parents, filling out a crib card with the baby's measurements and attaching a lock of hair to it, and giving parents the baby's blanket (Stewart, 1993). Such small acts of caring are long remembered, and help grieving family months—even years—later.

Always focus on cultural strengths, not perceived weaknesses. Says Linda Bolton: "I do not believe that one can become an expert of a different culture, but we can ask, 'How do we differ and how are we similar and what can we learn from each other?'" (Morrison, 1991-92, p. 14). And so often in the asking we discover that we have more similarities than differences.

STAFF RIGHTS AND WORKPLACE ETHICS

"When my brother began medical school," remembers a new nursing clinical instructor, "they shook the hand of each future physician and crooned, 'Welcome Doctor.' But the first day at my new job, they announced to the nursing students: 'At the end of the semester, a third of you will be gone.' I looked around the room and wondered, *Why are nurses so hard on each other? Why can't we treat our students and coworkers with the same respect, flexibility, and room for individual differences that we accord our patients? How can we expect nurses to value the rights of their patients when they, themselves, don't feel valued? Nurses have rights, too.*"

The JCAHO (1994, p. 52) says that organizations should have "established policies and mechanisms that address any request by a staff member not to participate in an aspect of patient care, including treatment." Such situations include when cultural values or religious beliefs are in conflict, but are not meant to be an "out" for employees. "If a patient is especially complex or challenging," says a surgical I.C.U. nurse, "we make changes in assignments to support the staff so they aren't caring for the same patient 10 days in a row." Not only is this an example of being attuned to staff rights, it also helps to preserve patient rights.

Here's a four-way test of workplace ethics that might well guide our communication with other professionals: Is it true? Is it fair to all involved? Will it foster a spirit of caring about each other and the profession? Will it be helpful to everyone? All we have to give to our patients is who we are. And so much of who we are begins in the way we treat our coworkers.

AREN'T RELIGION AND SPIRITUALITY THE SAME?

The more technological healthcare becomes, the more intense the cravings of the human spirit. As Pierre Teilhard De Chardin eloquently said: "We are not human beings having a spiritual experience. We are spiritual beings having a human experience." When addressing a patient's spiritual needs, take a minute to ask yourself, "Am I meeting their needs or my own?" (Messner & Ward, 1989).

Beth, a nurse in the early stages of multiple sclerosis, attended a healing service at a local church, and returned to her job eager to share her experience with a paralyzed patient. *If Mr. James can just feel some of the hope and joy that I do,* she convinced herself as she immersed him in the whirlpool tub with a prayer and a loud affirmation. But the emotionally charged seasons of illness or death are never the right time to try to convert someone to your own belief system, no matter how well intended the gesture.

Patients experiencing serious illness frequently rely on faith to help them cope (Lazarus, 1980). Support what has meaning for them, even if it vastly differs from your own belief system. Take time to understand a patient's need for prayer or communion before surgery. "Staying with the patient and family," says Di Sarcini (1991, p. 23), "is a significant form of spiritual care. It says to the person and their family, 'I care; you are loved, supported, and important.'"

DID SOMEONE JUMP TO CONCLUSIONS?

Some people, it seems, get their only exercise jumping to conclusions. "When my grandmother was admitted with abdominal pain and distention," remembers a nurse, "they wheeled her down the hall where I was passing meds, and announced: 'Here's old Mrs. Matthews with her usual complaints.' She'd never been a patient in that hospital before, and I shudder to think those were some of the final words she heard before she slipped into a coma."

A patient with Crohn's disease made this comment: "People—even healthcare workers—are always saying to me, '*You're* sick? Well, you look fine to me, and you're able to go to the mall.' What they don't realize is that I'm too ill to get out of bed for days at a time. And, before I can go to the mall, I must know where all the restrooms are in case I have an attack of explosive diarrhea. Sometimes I think it would be easier if I had an arm or leg missing. Then people would know at a glance that something is wrong with me."

PAIN MANAGEMENT

One of the ways patients judge nursing care is by assistance with pain, both direct (administering an analgesic) and indirect (modifying a procedure to minimize discomfort) (Brown, 1986). "Many patients don't receive adequate pain control," notes an oncologist, "and I think that's because we tend to administer analgesics based on what *we* believe the patient needs. The problem with pain is that people can't see it."

Here's one easy-to-remember clinical approach to pain assessment and management:

Ask about pain regularly.
Assess pain systematically.

Believe the patient and family in their reports of pain and what relieves it.

Choose pain control options appropriate for the patient, family, and setting.

Deliver interventions in a timely, logical, and coordinated fashion.

Empower patients and their families.

> Enable them to control their course to the greatest extent possible. (U.S. Department of Health and Human Services, 1994, p. 24)

How many times have you heard a nurse or a doctor remark, "That post-op shouldn't be having that much pain" or "Oh, come on, it doesn't hurt that bad." Yet what a patient has to say about pain should be the primary source of our nursing pain assessment. Pain control is an important patient rights issue, and is an area where nursing can assume a leadership role.

"We cared for a patient with bone cancer in our office who carried around his pain like a camper with a back pack," recalls a nurse. "It never left him. I requested a consultation with our entire office team, and we came up with a plan for pain control that really worked. It was wonderful seeing his quality of life improve . . . he actually got to enjoy the holiday season with his visiting grandchildren. But more than that, it helped our office staff work better together to avoid making assumptions and judgments. We realized from his experience that, in the past, we tended to avoid patients we couldn't cure. I think in the future we'll be more confident and caring in the area of pain control in our terminally ill patients."

"Keep in mind that patients are often unable to abstractly define pain," says a hospice nurse. "If you ask them to rate their pain on a scale of 1 to 10, however, they can usually give you a good self-assessment of their pain."

Restraints and Other Protective Devices

Patients have the legal right to the least restrictive means of treatment, as well as a right to be cared for in a safe and dignified manner. There are times, however, when the use of physical restraint becomes necessary and nurses must balance these issues to provide the best possible patient care. Restraints and other protective devices should always be used with compassion and sensitivity. Remember that restraints can promote safety, but they can also compromise a patient's psychosocial integrity, limit movement and circulation, and increase vulnerability and powerlessness.

Discovering a loved one in restraints can be extremely distressing for the family. "After my father's stroke, he was hospitalized for several weeks," remembers Ella. "One morning my mother and a neighbor walked into his room only to find him tied to the bed frame with his gown up around his waist. Mama went into hysterics, shook her fist at Daddy's favorite nurse, and yelled: 'I thought this was a hospital—not a jail.' We later found out that he'd gotten confused during the night, pulled all his tubes out, climbed over the bed rails, and fallen on the floor. It was fortunate he didn't break a leg."

While restraints are sometimes clinically justified, they should never be used as a punitive measure, as a substitute for good nursing care, or as a convenience for nursing or medical staff. If a patient must be restrained, preserve their rights and dignity by being attentive to their circulation, skin integrity, hydration, nutrition, elimination, hygiene, and emotional needs.

Ask Me What I Think

People in today's consumer-driven society want more than ever to be involved in decisions regarding their care. Healthcare is not something done *to* them, but rather *with* them. If we fail to accomplish this, feelings of learned hopelessness, a "What's the use?" mentality, may ensue. A family member remarked to other visitors in the hospital coffee shop about her teen-age son who was injured in a motorcycle accident: "I'm not going to fuss with the nurses anymore. I just want Billy to get the best of care, and whenever I interfere, they just take it out on him."

Words can soften the most anxious of moments. "When they had to put me in isolation for possible tuberculosis," says Bette, "I was remembering when they carried my grandmother off to a sanitarium. I still have a bracelet she made for me there. My nurse just slapped an isolation sign on my door and didn't say a word to me. I cried for an hour. Couldn't she have said something?"

Educator Marge Funk takes a patient-centered, ethical approach when teaching her students the art and science of critical care. While mentoring them in the high-tech aspects of nursing, she underscores the need to truly focus on the patient. One way she accomplishes this is to include patients in all conversations, if possible, so they don't feel like educational exhibits. And she also requests permission to introduce a student into their care (Gordon, 1994).

PATIENT SATISFACTION SURVEYS

Investigating and trying to resolve a patient's complaint is another patient right (JCAHO, 1994). Patient satisfaction surveys often identify complaints as well as other opportunities for improvement. The feedback from these surveys is valuable in determining patient perceptions of an organization's care and services. Yet confidentiality of customer satisfaction surveys is also a patient right, and patients should always understand that information expressed will not affect the quality of future care. Many institutions make self-identification optional (Nelson & Niederberger, 1990), while others don't include a space for the patient's name at all.

HELP ME MAINTAIN MY INDEPENDENCE

Nurses have the unique function of assisting patients to maximize independence through health maintenance, recovery from illness, or a peaceful death, depending on the circumstances.

"We once cared for a terminally ill patient who desperately wanted to die at home," remembers a patient discharge coordinator. "But I'd been in that home, and while it was safe, I knew that she could receive better services in a nursing home. The bottom line was the patient felt she could be more independent and peaceful in her home environment. So we taught her daughters to care for her. She passed away after spending the morning around the kitchen table having coffee with her family. When she drew her last breath, her poodle was dozing on a quilt at the foot of her bed."

WHAT MAKES A PATIENT A PERSON?

"I love beautiful presents and I rarely give a gift without wrapping it up in lovely paper, tied up with a festive bow," says Amy, a nursing student who just completed a clinical rotation at a homeless shelter. "I guess that's why I was surprised when one of the best lessons of my life wasn't wrapped up in a pretty package. It arrived on a cold, snowy December morning dressed in a torn, thin coat, wearing frayed gloves with two of the fingers out. That man hadn't been able to buy his medicine for several years and he asked me to check his blood pressure. There was only one chair in the little room where we keep the equipment. He motioned for me to sit down, and said it was no bother for him to stand. When I insisted he take the seat, a tear trickled down his nearly frozen cheek. I'll never forget that moment ... it's when I learned that behind every patient is real human being."

I learned a similar lesson when I was doing some consultation work at a nursing home. The Director of Nursing stacked several charts on a conference room table, all belonging to patients with the same strain of infection. I immediately recognized the "UTI in 21B" as one of my elementary school teachers; she'd been in a comatose state for six months. I shared with the staff classroom memories of the day the Beatles made their first appearance on the Ed Sullivan Show. My teacher had been so sure the world was coming to an end with "that kind of music" being played, and kept stressing how important it was to her that we all grow up to be responsible people. We all had a good chuckle, but they began to see her as a real person—a teacher—after that.

Patients are people. Maybe that frail gentleman whose daughter told you through tears that "Dad got old overnight" was once a vibrant husband, father, community leader. And the ICU patient, stripped on admission of all earthly possessions and now garbed in a gown that says "HOSPITAL PROPERTY," may have once supervised the nursery at her church. Take time to admire family photos displayed on a bedside table, and ask their loved ones about their memories of them. Remember, your patients have a past.

BE AN ADVOCATE

A young lady who underwent a trigeminal nerve block for intractable facial pain describes this harrowing experience: "There was such a casual disregard for patient comfort during what was an extremely uncomfortable procedure. They were too busy 'talking' the resident through the procedure to pay much attention to me. One technician who recognized how miserable I was hugged me, and I really appreciated that. I feel it should be second nature for healthcare providers to function as patient advocates and prevent needless suffering."

Of all the personnel that patients must deal with during a hospital stay, nurses spend more time with patients, are more aware of their needs, and are their greatest advocates. Consumer groups are dispensing information like never before to educate healthcare customers about their rights as patients and how to determine if they're receiving quality care (Martin, 1993). Today's patients are better informed, have clearer expectations, and are more assertive. Patient-centered care, which consciously considers the customer's perspective, is gaining rapid momentum in healthcare, and represents an important nursing advocacy strategy. Experts stress: "Advocacy must be a process, not an event. Nurses must constantly ask patients and families what they need" (Gordon, 1994, p. 6).

Nurses function as patient advocates in a number of ways that impact satisfaction with care. When a patient doesn't receive adequate information before being asked to sign a consent, for instance, we advocate for additional information so that they're indeed able to give informed consent. We make referrals so a patient's concerns about advance directives are adequately addressed. We avoid the use of restraints when possible by instituting alternative measures (locating patients at risk for falls close to the nurses' station, assessing their environment for risk factors, providing patient/family education about safety).

ETHICAL DILEMMAS

Contemporary nurses are often confronted with situations that require ethical decision making. Ethics is concerned with the study of moral standards, judgments, choices, values, beliefs, and problems. Ethics as defined by McFadden is the assessment of the morality of human acts through the critical process of natural reason (Applegate, 1993).

When facing an ethical dilemma, nurses may feel ambivalent. Conflicting beliefs and values often prevent clear-cut answers. It is important to be aware that our personal values, attitudes, and beliefs influence our decision-making process. Being familiar with nursing and JCAHO standards, and how they apply to clinical practice, can help in dealing with ethical considerations. Using an interdisciplinary team approach can clarify issues and strengthen decisions.

The JCAHO (1994) states that organizations should have a mechanism for addressing ethical issues. Susan, a nurse who sits on the ethics committee of a large metropolitan hospital, says: "In nursing, we are often overwhelmed and confused and in conflict with dilemmas in our practice." She points out that when such questions arise, the first step is to determine whether the concern is an ethical, clinical, policy, or legal issue.

Consider the case of Minnie, an 85-year-old patient who was in relatively good health until she slipped on the ice going to bingo and fractured her hip. On admission, her husband (and durable power of attorney for healthcare), gave the physician a copy of her living will. "I don't want to be hooked up to any of those machines and be a burden to my family," Minnie said in a voice as fragile as a china teacup. "Everett and I have enough to make ends meet, but nothing extra."

But in the Post Anesthesia Care Unit following the surgical repair of her hip, Minnie went into respiratory distress and was placed on a ventilator. Three weeks later, when she was barely responsive and unable to be weaned from the ventilator, Everett asked the physician to discontinue it.

"Take me off the case," Max, a registered nurse in the SICU, demanded. "My church doesn't believe like that. She didn't get a chance. I was brought up to believe all life is sacred. What if she could have recovered and you denied her that?" Max even crossed the professional line to let his opinion be known to Minnie's family.

After a night of agonizing, Everett stayed true to his wife's original wishes. The law in Minnie's state allows advance directives to be followed. But the incident brought to light a number of pertinent issues involving staff and patient rights and legal implications, later discussed at the SICU staff meeting and Medical Center Ethics Committee. Because of the institution's policy of respecting personnel's religious convictions, Max was permitted to withdraw from the case. But in a private meeting, the unit manager reminded Max, an otherwise superb critical care nurse, that it's not appropriate to impose your personal value system on others. For in order for patients and families to be satisfied with overall care, they need to be supported in their beliefs whenever it's legally feasible.

Nurses interact with patients on a more intimate level than any other healthcare workers, and are often there during a moment of crisis or a significant life event (Messner & Ward, 1989). When registered nurses were asked to identify their primary ethical concerns, the top six responses were: rationing of healthcare, end-of-life decisions, abortions, advance directives, assisted suicide, and euthanasia (Epstein, 1994, p. 15).

"Many ethical issues can be anticipated," emphasizes a unit manager, "but in our stress we often don't ask enough questions. For example, a patient may say they want 'everything' done. We can assume a preventive stance by identifying what 'everything' means to them and by using language that means the same thing to everyone involved." When an ethical issue in a patient's care arises, both patient and family should be advised, as appropriate, on how to access the ethics committee and the ethical issue resolution process.

THE FINAL DAYS OF LIFE

Sometimes we forget the awesome beauty that acceptance of adversity can bring to a life. The right of a patient to be an individual until life's final moment is poignantly expressed by Mal Warshaw, who photographed terminally ill patients for Elisabeth Kübler-Ross' book, *To Live Until We Say Goodbye* (1992, p. 8). He writes: "I noted the faces of people who have a terminal disease, and who have come to terms with their own impending death, have a look that is a marvelous combination of tranquility and incredible power and insight."

The emotional, physical, and spiritual preparation for death can be a time of transformation . . . through remembering, growth, and peaceful completion of this life (Kolkmeier, 1995). Such patients frequently emerge as new people, affirms Dr. Kübler-Ross. Free from the trivial struggles that limit the healthy, they often exude a creativity that far surpasses human capabilities, personal expectations, or educational preparation. While there can be no curing without caring, there *can* be caring without curing (Leininger, 1981).

To ensure compassionate, thoughtful care for patients facing the end of life, take a close look at issues of comfort, dignity, symptom management, culture, and spirituality. This presents an extraordinary opportunity for helping the patient experience peace of mind and spirit in the process of dying.

JUST BE THERE

"Presence," writes Anne Di Sarcini (1991, p. 23), "is so powerful that it defies definition." Often we underestimate the power of just being there for our patients. The quiet acceptance of people as individuals communicates volumes about how much we value them. That presence is a part of all that is nursing. "Persons who are studying to become registered nurses are not simply learning an occupation," write Ellis and Hartley (1980, p. vii), "They are 'becoming' nurses in the most profound sense of the word. To themselves, their families, and their communities they will be nurses wherever they are."

It all boils down to this: people look to nurses to respect and protect their rights. Patient satisfaction (and our own satisfaction) with the changing healthcare system largely depends on our continuing to earn that trust. Although sometimes intangible, it's one of the best rewards in nursing.

References

American Hospital Association. (1992). *Patient's Bill of Rights.* Chicago: Author.

Applegate, M. I. (1993). Ethics. In J. M. Black and E. Matassarin-Jacobs (Eds.), *Luckmann & Sorensen's medical-surgical nursing* (4th ed.). Philadelphia: W. B. Saunders Company.

Bailey, I. (1985). View from the horizontal side of caring. *Nursing 85, 15*(10), 53.

Brown, L. (1986). The experience of care: Patient perspectives. *Topics in Clinical Nursing, 8*(2), 56-62.

Buechner, F. (1993). *Wishful thinking.* New York: Harper Collins Publishers.

Cabell Huntington Hospital. (1995). Patient rights and responsibilities. *Cabell Huntington Hospital patient handbook* (pp. 12-14). Huntington, WV: Author.

DiSarcini, A. (1991). Spiritual care at a code. *Journal of Christian Nursing, 8*(3), 20-23.

Dossey, B. M., & Keegan, L. (1995). Self-assessments: Facilitating healing in self and others. In B.M. Dossey, L. Keegan, C.E. Guzzetta, and L.G. Kolkmeier (Eds.), *Holistic nursing* (pp. 219-237). Gaithersburg, MD: Aspen Publishers, Inc.

Ellis, J. R., & Hartley, C. L. (1980). *Nursing in today's world.* Philadelphia: J.B. Lippincott Co.

Epstein, D. (1994). What RNs identify as their most pressing ethical concerns. *RN, 57*(8), 15.

Ethics. (1993). *Rural Nurse Connection, 1*(3), 1-2.

Frawley, K. A. (1994). Confidentiality in the computer age. *RN, 57*(7), 59-60.

Gerteis, M., Edgman-Levitan, S., Daley, J., & Delbanco, T. L. (Eds.). (1993). *Through the patient's eyes: Understanding and promoting patient-centered care.* San Francisco: Jossey-Bass Inc., Publishers.

Gordon, S. (1994, June). Inside the patient-driven system. *Critical Care Nurse* (supplement), 2-28.

JCAHO. (1994). *The Joint Commission 1995 accreditation manual for hospitals. Volume I: Standards.* Oakbrook Terrace, IL: Author.

Johnson, S., & Wilson, L. (1984). *The one minute sales person.* New York: Avon Books.

Kolkmeier, L. G. (1995). Self-reflection: Consulting the truth within. In B.M. Dossey, L. Keegan, C.E. Guzzetta, and L.G. Kolkmeier (Eds.), *Holistic nursing: A handbook for practice* (2nd ed., pp. 335-363). Gaithersburg, MD: Aspen Publishers, Inc.

Koska, M. T. (1992, Nov. 5). Surveying customer needs, not satisfaction, is crucial to CQI. *Hospitals,* 50-53.

Kübler-Ross, E., & Warshaw, M. (1992). *To live until we say goodbye.* New York: Simon & Shuster.

Lazarus, R. S. (1980). The stress and coping paradigm. In L. Bonde and J. C. Rosen (Eds.), *Competence and coping during adulthood* (pp. 28-69). Hanover, NH: University Press of New England.

Leininger, M. M. (1981). *Caring: An essential human need. Proceedings of the three national caring conferences.* Thorofare, NJ: Charles B. Slack, Inc.

Lewis, S. J., & Morton, G. B. (1994). Psychosocial assessment. In Bolander, J.R. (Ed.), *Sorensen and Luckmann's basic nursing—A psychophysiologic approach* (3rd ed., pp. 627-674). Philadelphia: W.B. Saunders Co.

Lipkin, G. B., & Cohen, R. G. (1992). *Effective approaches to patients' behavior.* New York: Springer Publishing Co.

Long, C. O., & Greeneich, D. S. (1994). Family satisfaction techniques: Meeting family expectations. *Dimensions in Critical Care Nursing, 13,* 104-111.

Martin, J. (1993, Nov.) The new way to take charge of your healthcare. *McCalls,* 48-55.

Messner, R. L., & Ward, D. (1989). In S. Lewis, R. D. Knowles-Grainger, W. A. McDowell, R. J. Gregory, & R. L. Messner (Eds.), *Manual of psychosocial nursing interventions* (pp. 259-269). Philadelphia: W. B. Saunders Co.

Milholland, D. K. (1994). Privacy and confidentiality of patient information. *Journal of Nursing Administration, 24*(2), 19-24.

Morrison, S. (1991-92, Winter). Nursing unlimited. *Graduating Nurse (Minorities Issue),* 14.

Mount, B. (1993, Jan./Feb.). Whole person care: Beyond psychological and physical needs. *The American Journal of Hospice and Palliative Care,* 28-37.

Nelson, C. W., & Niederberger, J. (1990). Patient satisfaction surveys: An opportunity for total quality improvement. *Hospital and Health Services Administration, 35*(3), 409-427.

Press, Ganey Associates, Inc. (1992). *The satisfaction report.* South Bend, IN: Author.

Press, I. (1984, April). The predisposition to file claims: The patient's perspective. *Law, Medicine and Health Care,* 53-62.

Schiff, R. L., Goldberg, D., & Ansell, D. A. (1992). Access to health care. In R. P. Wenzel, *Assessing quality health care* (pp. 139-155). Baltimore: Williams & Wilkins.

Spitzer, R. B. (1988). Meeting customer expectations. *Nursing Administration Quarterly, 12*(3), 31-39.

Stewart, J. F. (1993, Sept./Oct.). Letter to the editor. *Physician,* 23.

Tanenbaum, R., & Berman, M. (1993, April). Why even patients who like you will sue you for malpractice. *Physician's Management,* 85-97.

U. S. Department of Health and Human Services. (1994, March). *Management of cancer pain* (Clinical Practice Guideline #9). Rockville, MD: U. S. Department of Health and Human Services, Public Health Service, Agency for Health Care Policy and Research.

Woolhandler, S., & Himmelstein, D. U. (1989). Resolving the cost/access conflict: The case for a national health program. *Journal of General Internal Medicine, 4,* 54-60.

Chapter 5

PATIENT EDUCATION

A Key to Increased Satisfaction

Education is a social process. . . Education is growth. . . Education is
preparation for life; education is life itself.
— John Dewey (Connor, 1992, p.1)

In the course of a lifetime, we hear millions of words. What makes some of them take up residence in our hearts and minds yet others fall by the wayside? And how can we as nurses speak memorable words, especially when it comes to patient education, one of the most important and long-lasting services we provide?

According to the Joint Commission on Accreditation for Healthcare Organizations (JCAHO), the goal of educating the patient, and/or when appropriate, family, is "to improve patient health outcomes by promoting recovery, speeding return to function, promoting healthy behavior, and appropriately involving the patient in his or her care decisions." Education should:

- facilitate the understanding of the patient's health status, healthcare options, and consequences of options selected;

- encourage participation in the decision-making process about healthcare options;

- increase the potential to follow the therapeutic health care plan for patient;

- maximize care skills;

- increase the ability to cope with health status/prognosis/outcome;

- enhance continuing care; and

- promote a healthy patient lifestyle. (JCAHO, 1994, p. 189)

Today, patient education is no longer the sole responsibility of nursing, but should be planned and provided in concert with other disciplines to assure consistency and continuity.

Today's consumers are increasingly well informed, and most expect a more active involvement in their healthcare. Healthcare consumers want procedures explained to them and at least an attempt at least made to answer their questions (Spitzer, 1988). All too often, however, nurses lack confidence in their own abilities to provide effective patient education (Rankin & Stallings, 1990). Yet research indicates that patients who receive adequate education have shorter hospital stays, experience fewer complications and less distress, and are more satisfied with their healthcare experience in general (Padberg & Padberg, 1990).

Information is a key to making more informed choices (Bader, 1988; Lucas, Morris, & Alexander, 1988). With patients being discharged from the hospital sooner, and more acute care taking place in outpatient and home settings, this presents a particular challenge and opportunity for nurses (Rega, 1993). Providing effective patient education not only leads to better clinical outcomes and more healthy behaviors; it also saves healthcare dollars by cutting down on preventable problems, and decreases readmissions and outpatient visits.

Education changes a person for all time, whether they remember the specific content or not. Still, the value of time-intensive patient education must be weighed against all the other pressing concerns on a busy nurse's "TO DO" list. Here are some arguments we've heard from nurses:

- "Patient education takes too much time. I have enough to do already, and it's really not my job."

- "The only reason we do patient education is to satisfy JCAHO. Once they come and go, we'll fall right back into the same habit of doing nothing."

- "You teach patients until you're blue in the face. No one remembers any of that stuff. They're going to do what they want to do anyway."

- "That patient's had diabetes for years. He knows everything he needs to know."

- "I never get any feedback as to whether my patient education actually helped anyone."

- "Patients don't listen to us. They pay more attention to their family and friends."

- "Patients always ask me questions when I'm busy passing meds or in the middle of a treatment."

- "I think I've made a difference. Then, I find out my patient was just acting like they understood in order to please me."

- "   "

(I left an extra space so that you, the reader, can add an additional frustration you've encountered.)

There's an old proverb that says if you give a person a fish, you feed them for a day. But if you teach that person to fish, you feed them for a lifetime. When we teach our patients, we invest in a future of better health for them.

Here are some secrets to more effective patient education. They can be easily applied to any clinical setting.

TAKE TIME TO ESTABLISH RAPPORT

It really is true: people don't care what you know until they know that you care. Begin by finding out what your patient cares about most. Setting the tone with a warm, friendly, comforting atmosphere, you can then switch gears to the more mechanical, procedural approach when your patient is ready.

Social conversation serves a purpose. It sets the tone for the whole healthcare encounter, and helps to establish trust, and rapport. People are generally more comfortable with someone they perceive to be like them in some way. "Sit a spell," as they say in Appalachia, and establish some common ground. First things first, especially if you're an outsider. When you've shown a genuine interest in the things that matter most to your patients, helping them to discover their unique worth, they'll sense your approval and naturally open up to you.

Once when I was working with a group of clinic patients who had tuberculosis, I learned that some of them were also visiting a local folk healer. I decided to pay him a call myself, and I learned firsthand about the incorrect information my patients were receiving. I also learned that the folk healer, a very charismatic man, had mastered the art of rapport. And that he, not I, held them in the palm of his hand.

So often we talk without really communicating. If you're a nurse in your early twenties, and you're trying to teach a middle-aged male who is having difficulty accepting a new diagnosis of prostate cancer, just be honest: "I've never experienced what you're going through, but I really want to help. If you were in my shoes, what would you say to me right now?" But always be true to your own personality. If you are naturally more business-like in your approach, that's okay.

It's a well-known fact in the world of hospitals that patients talk more to the housekeeping personnel than they do to medical and nursing staff. The sad truth is, people do confide in the lady who asks sympathetically as she mops the floor: "I saw that look on your face when you tried to get out of bed. You can tell me, honey . . . how are you *really* doing?"

People long for personalized attention. As basic as it seems, they love the sound of their own name. Call patients by their name and use it often. That's part of teaching the whole person. And don't forget to communicate what nurses are all about, too. The media has tried to tell the public what to think of us. Yet as one patient expressed after his nurse had spent several sessions educating him about his new ostomy, "You nurses are Jacks and Jills of all trades. I never knew that before." Part of setting the groundwork for future rapport is to educate consumers about the many facets of our roles.

APPRECIATE AGE-RELATED DIFFERENCES

"When I was being scheduled for outpatient oral surgery, I inquired as to whether the staff had been trained in CPR," remembers a patient. "My dentist very good naturedly escorted me on a tour and said: 'We have a system here that works rather well. We treat the adults like children and the children like adults.'"

Humorous perhaps in the retelling, we as nurses ofttimes falsely assume that adults and children learn in essentially the same manner. There are, however, some very striking differences. Age-related nuances are receiving increased attention from the Joint Commission, who expect nurses to demonstrate age-related competencies for the specific populations they serve. Children are not merely small grownups; they have a shorter attention span than adults, and need a great deal of affirmation. Patient education for this population is often best accomplished through play. The child's developmental level should always be taken into consideration to determine the best approach for presenting information.

At the other end of the spectrum are the elderly, America's fastest growing population. They have a wealth of life experiences to build on, but they are typically more hesitant than younger adults. "It's not uncommon for an elderly patient to proceed with the caution of a preschooler crossing a busy street when presented with new information," observes a gerontologist. "They look both ways for signs of danger before going forward." The elderly often have difficulty understanding complex sentences and abstract concepts as well—sometimes even the gist of a story (Rankin & Stallings, 1990). When teaching the elderly, take time to assess their sensory deficits and level of cognitive functioning, and adapt your teaching plan to identified needs. Speak slowly in a clear, low-pitched tone of voice, using short, simple sentences and concrete language. When repeating information, avoid varying the terminology. Document techniques proven to be effective to guide other caregivers in providing and reinforcing your patient education (DeVos, 1989).

FIND OUT WHAT THE PATIENT EXPECTS

One of the greatest fears patients experience is in not knowing what lies ahead of them. Yet patient expectations are always a key to satisfaction. In one study, for example, most of the patients interviewed wanted to receive pre-operative education from a surgeon because they considered him to be the most reliable source of information. In the same study, a number of subjects commented that they preferred to receive information concerning anesthesia directly from the anesthetist (Leino-Kilpi & Vuorenheimo, 1993).

Other researchers found that nearly half of outpatients desire more illness information. Subjects were significantly more satisfied with their treatment than with the information they received (Harris, 1992). One way to assess what patients expect and to promote more realistic expectations is to provide them with an informational pamphlet or initiate phone contact with prospective customers prior to their contact with your agency.

Don't fall into the trap of assuming you know what the patient wants. Sometimes our own education gets in the way of what's best for a particular patient. Always be a student. Terminally ill patients, for instance, may greatly benefit from education so they can make more informed choices about pain control—even though their life expectancy may be short. Knowing these expectations helps to plan meaningful education with the entire care team.

DETERMINE HOW YOUR PATIENT LEARNS BEST

"If you discover how a patient learns best, you can teach them almost anything," advises a wonderfully caring physician who himself has a learning disability. Determine if your patient watches TV and videos, spends long hours at the computer, enjoys reading, or talks over problems with family or friends. This will give you clues as to whether they process information by hearing, by seeing, or through feelings, and will help you plan more personalized patient education activities. Some medical centers now have reference libraries and closed circuit TV programs for patients and families.

Keep in mind that a combination of teaching methods (involving as many senses as feasible) will create a more lasting impression. Let them see it, feel it, touch it, hear it. But take into consideration any sensory obstacles a patient might have.

"They acted like I was just another Joe Blow who didn't know beans," remembers a factory worker. "Finally, they did hand me a pamphlet, but no one took the time to answer my questions. I like to talk things out." Pamphlets are fine as an adjunct to the human connection in education. But the thing that will last is what you place in a person's heart, not merely his or her hands.

START EARLY

Begin patient education planning prior to admission, if possible, or on the day of admission (Rankin & Stallings, 1990; Tirk, 1992), starting with the initial nursing assessment. Baseline data such as education and literacy levels, primary language, living conditions, coping skills, cultural and religious practices, motivation, and conditions likely to influence a patient's ability to practice self-care (e.g., physical and cognitive limitations) will give you valuable information and identify important concerns and barriers to learning (JCAHO, 1994). Caring, open-ended questions will usually elicit the most meaningful responses.

Patients who must digest large amounts of highly technical information are particular candidates for early teaching, especially in these days of shortened hospital stays (Padberg & Padberg,

1990). Louise, a staff nurse in an inner-city health clinic, says, "I often think of myself as a translator. The doctor speaks with the patient in complex, medical terminology. Afterwards, I have to translate his message into plain, everyday words the patient can understand." A well-informed patient (who is not overloaded with information) is more likely to be a partner in care with nurses and other providers (Harris, 1992).

One study of ambulatory surgery patients revealed patient dissatisfaction with the timeliness of information presented (Inguanzo & Harju, 1985). Patients clearly want information early on, and those who are satisfied with this important aspect of care are more likely to return for future services (Pica-Furey, 1993). There should be few, if any, surprises when a patient leaves your clinic or office setting, or at the time of hospital discharge. Never try to instruct a patient on their way out the door.

BEGIN WITH WHAT THE PATIENT ALREADY KNOWS

This is one of the most basic principles of how adults learn best, for it gives patients a confident edge, puts them at ease, and increases the likelihood of success (Morgan & Philp, 1985). Unlike children, adults learn by building on past life lessons (Gessner, 1983). In fact, adults actually define themselves through their experiences.

Vernon Sanders once observed, "Experience is a hard teacher because she gives the test first, the lesson afterwards" (Mason, 1993, p. 32). Use examples from the rich reservoir of the patient's own life story, if at all possible. Stroke their strengths, and compare and contrast the familiar and the unfamiliar to give patients a feeling of more control.

Jesus recognized the value of this when he taught people through parables. In short, he met them right where they were, and built on their knowledge base. If you're teaching a dairy farmer how to give himself an injection, recognize his experience in administering antibiotics to his cattle. One astute patient with a third-grade education commented: "You don't have to be in Who's Who to know what's what. It's not your book learning that makes you smart; it's your powers to reason." There's a lot of wisdom in that statement.

Affirm family strengths as well, and tap into their rich reservoir of expertise to promote involvement in the patient's continuing healthcare plan. When instructing a patient's curious engineer son about home total parenteral nutrition therapy, for instance, take time to delve into a little more detail when explaining how the IV pump works.

As Flannery O'Connor once said, "Storytelling is an attempt to make someone who doesn't want to listen, listen, and who doesn't want to see, see" (Hemley, 1994). If you want to reach others, you do it by being specific. A story is the shortest path between two souls.

In the Appalachian culture, storytelling is a big part of learning. "I've found that you can weave complex nursing concepts into the fabric of patients' lives as they spin a yarn," explains an experienced nurse educator who works in a rural clinic.

"One of my patients is a groomer at the horse farm that's raised two Kentucky Derby winners," says a nurse practitioner. "He'd lost his spleen in a car accident and was particularly at risk for pneumococcal pneumonia, and last fall I was trying to convince him to take the vaccine. 'I'm only 43,' he countered. 'I believe I'll wait.' I admired the pictures of his horses, then said, 'You know, postponing your pneumonia shot is like closing the barn door after the horses get out.' He chuckled softly and answered, 'I guess you've got a point there.' He not only changed his mind on the pneumonia vaccine, but decided to take the flu vaccine as well."

Before beginning any teaching, it's essential to adequately (albeit sometimes discreetly) assess a patients' knowledge of the subject matter, as well as their educational and literacy levels. If they tell you they "can't see the words because they left their glasses at home" or that "your handwriting is much prettier than mine," these may be pieces of the puzzle to a literacy problem.

Recognize that Knowledge Is Power

It does our patients no favor to keep them in the dark and intrigued with the mystique of the medical world (Jones, 1983). One of the ways we empower our patients, and build their confidence and control, is by debunking their myths and misconceptions. Sound patient education increases a patient's options. Yet don't assume that even a healthcare professional understands everything. "When I had my M.I.," remembers one patient, "I heard them say, 'He's a cardiac cath tech; he knows everything.' I may have known it in theory, but not as a patient." And the same goes for the patient who's had ulcerative colitis for 20 years. Experience with an illness isn't necessarily synonymous with expertise.

Don't Minimize Patient Concerns

Remembers one patient: "I'd been on birth control pills for 10 years straight and asked my OB/GYN doctor what would happen if I discontinued them. He answered with a shrug, 'Well, you could bleed to death. Two women did.' Then he left me sobbing."

Another patient recounts the time she went to her doctor thinking she might have an ovarian cyst. She'd seen a TV program about ovarian disease and thought she'd better get her symptoms checked out. After he examined her, he said, "You might have cancer. Go home for a month and don't worry about it, and we'll evaluate things again then."

Take time to really understand a patient's perceptions in light of the total picture. If they have just received bad news or are experiencing a difficult adjustment period, for instance, this will profoundly affect their assimilation of information. Find out what your cancer patient has heard via the grapevine about the side effects of chemotherapy. You may be surprised that they are dreading complications that are highly unlikely.

SAVE THE MOST SENSITIVE ISSUES FOR LAST

Issues involving money and other highly personal areas, for instance, can make patients wonder, "Why would a nurse need to know that?" Yet money is often at the root of seeming disinterest or non-compliance. "Them little pills is a hundred bucks a whack!" a gentleman at the drugstore commented as he counted out money for his new prescription. Chances are, if it comes down to putting food on the table and paying the utility bill, he'll think twice about having it refilled, unless he's really convinced of the benefit.

ELIMINATE ENVIRONMENTAL DISTRACTIONS

Noise, poor ventilation or lighting, an uncomfortable temperature, and lack of privacy will negatively affect your teaching efforts. Adult patients are generally used to having some degree of control over their personal environment and will quickly become distracted or annoyed if they're physically uncomfortable.

DON'T FORGET THE PATIENT'S FAMILY AND FRIENDS

A big part of veterinary medicine is interacting with the pet's owner. Likewise, professionals in the field of pediatrics spend considerable time fielding questions and gathering data from family members. Whatever the practice environment, the patient's significant others will influence them long after our instruction has ended. That's why experts say that one of the most important factors for successful patient education (both in the inpatient and home setting) is to keep all involved parties well informed (Moore & Komras, 1993). If patients' significant other(s) can't come to the hospital during the day, plan educational sessions for them during evening hours. Patient education is an around-the-clock activity.

Be sure to assess family dynamics and plan teaching that doesn't keep family members in the dark, yet doesn't violate patient confidentiality either. "I think my sister has a touch of pneumonia, but of course they never tell me anything," muses her only living relative. "I guess they have a lot of practice at that."

The JCAHO (1994, p. 191) says that "the patient and/or, when appropriate, his or her family (should be) provided with appropriate education and training to increase knowledge of the patient's illness and treatment needs, and to learn skills and behaviors that promote recovery and improve function." This information should be presented in a manner congruent with the family's level of understanding. Involving the family at an appropriate level helps to create a climate of trust, and breaks down invisible walls that may sabotage our best efforts. Furthermore, reduced trust in healthcare providers decreases the likelihood that patients will follow a therapeutic regimen and may predispose them to perceive actual harm (Press, Ganey, & Malone, 1991).

SCHEDULE PATIENT EDUCATION AROUND THE PATIENT'S NEEDS

A patient who is exhausted from having physical therapy or who is in pain or hungry is not in a prime state for learning. Timing is everything (Gessner, 1983). One patient who underwent podiatry surgery recalls: "They tried to tell me how to take care of my foot while they were jamming me with a needle." An overweight patient who just had her annual pap smear recalls: "They get you in those stirrups and then they try to talk to you about your weight."

BE OPEN TO THE UNEXPECTED

Seize the moment. If a prime opportunity for patient education arises during a bedbath or while ambulating a patient, don't hesitate to integrate patient education with other patient care activities if time permits.

Go with what is most meaningful for the patient at that particular time. Just as people are quickly frustrated with what they perceive as meaningless work, they also become turned off with information that appears to have little practical benefit for them. You can fill in details later on (Cunningham, 1993).

There's no time like the present. Look for teachable moments and be open to serendipity. "Always be prepared to revise your goals at a moment's notice," says a flight nurse. "That may seem like a daring departure from tradition, but it often saves you time in the long run." Besides, the patient will likely better remember the conversation if it occurs during an on-the-spot time when the two of you were connecting as individuals, where the nurse is truly present to the patient.

THINK CLARITY

The art of patient education is to make the complex simple, not the simple complex. In Bader's (1988) research on nursing care behaviors that predict patient satisfaction, the use of simple language was the best predictor of satisfaction with education. Keep it simple with handouts, too. A few key points, simple diagrams, and a telephone number to call back for questions is far superior to a grandiose handbook.

What is clear to us nurses can seem vague or downright confusing to our patients, especially after they leave the structured medical environment. Several years back, I coordinated an outpatient stool screening program to test for occult (or hidden) blood. One patient mailed back his specimen cards, unused, with this explanation: "I'm sorry I can't be a part of this. My religion prohibits me from dabbling in the occult."

PUT THE LESSON TO IMMEDIATE USE

Adults are very problem oriented and need to see that education is not an exercise in futility, but rather something which addresses a felt need or problem. Whenever possible, strive for immediate application. Some patients may tend to be passive. We are a society of spectators, who find it preferable to sit in front of the tube than to be actively involved. Our challenge is to convince our patients that what we are teaching will make a real difference in their lives.

INVOLVE THE PATIENT IN THE LEARNING PROCESS

The key to effective patient education is to figure out what the patient or family needs to know, then come up with a plan to make that happen. Like preparing a surface helps paint to adhere, your patient education has a better likelihood of sticking if you prepare. Adults learn better when they've helped to plan and actively participate in the educational session. Set learning goals with the patient, and think of yourself as a coach rather than an authority figure.

Patients have a personal responsibility in their own educational process, however. They should provide their caregivers with accurate and complete information about past and current problems; they are responsible for following the proposed treatment plan and for any adverse outcomes if they refuse prescribed treatment; and they are to respect an organization's rules and regulations as well as other patients and staff (JCAHO, 1994).

STEER AWAY FROM A CLASSROOM APPROACH

An informal, relaxing style is more conducive to spontaneity. Some adults may have performed poorly in school, and are very resistant to any setting that resembles learning "the three R's." For these individuals, a casual conference room setting, the privacy of their hospital room, or a quiet office usually works best. And don't forget the hospitality component. Being "the hostess with the mostest" really goes a long way toward showing you care enough to give your very best.

Yet still others may feel they "missed something" by not graduating from school. "You didn't spell my name right on my diploma," corrected a patient who had completed a six-week educational course on management of COPD. When the nurse rescripted his full name in beautiful calligraphy, he announced with a gap-toothed grin to a growing crowd: "I just might return for post-graduate work."

Our own mothers perfected a skill we can apply today. Look for opportunities to make life situations an informal classroom. It's well known that play is a child's work, and is where a lot of life's valuable lessons are learned. Adults can likewise learn during fun group activities. Let's say your nursing home patients are enjoying a birthday party for one of the residents. A patient pipes up and asks, "Can a diabetic have cake once a day?" You have an opportunity for a patient education moment.

COORDINATE THE CONTENT OF ALL PATIENT EDUCATION PROVIDED TO PROMOTE CONTINUITY

Even within the same professional discipline, we all approach patient education differently. Yet an organized interdisciplinary approach is crucial. If three nurses demonstrate wound care using different supplies, the patient will likely be confused. Collaborate with the entire interdisciplinary team to improve the likelihood that providers are reinforcing the same message. The more individuals who stress the same key points, the more important it will seem to the patient, too.

Part of patient advocacy is helping them coordinate their communication with other caregivers. Perhaps one of your office patients is anxious about a newly discovered lump in her breast. You notice her pacing in the waiting room, and know that it will be at least 15 minutes before the doctor can see her. Even if you're too pushed for time to sit down with her, you can offer her a note pad and suggest she begin to jot down some of her concerns so she won't be as intimidated or forget them when she sees the doctor.

DOCUMENTATION OF PATIENT EDUCATION

No discussion of continuity of care is complete without mentioning documentation. We've all heard the cliché: if it's not documented, it's not done. To that, one nurse jokes, "We have nurses

here who would rather have dental work done than to document."
Sadly, much of what nurses do is never reflected in the medical
record, and many nurses neither see documentation as a critical
part of total patient care nor believe that anyone needs or values
their entries (Parker, Wells, Buchanan, & Benjamin, 1994). Hence,
while it is essential to document pertinent aspects of patient education, nurses and other caregivers frequently provide superb
patient education without doing so.

Documentation, however, is critical for cost accounting.
Inadequate documentation may result in a loss of reimbursement
by third-party payers. An excellent place to begin is with the
JCAHO standards on patient education. "We developed a form at
our medical center, based on these standards, where everyone
charts their patient's assessed educational needs, abilities, readi-
ness to learn (including barriers to learning), the techniques used,
and patient/family responses," says a med-surg nurse. "It helps us
build on the education the doctors, dietitians, pharmacists, and
others have provided." It also ensures a more concerted approach
by the entire interdisciplinary team and keeps multiple caregivers
from posing the same questions, which is extremely frustrating to
patients. Such an educational plan should be initiated on admission for hospitalized patients, and carried out as appropriate for
their length of stay.

Still, don't let documentation dominate your practice. One surgeon says that healthcare has gotten to the place where "we do the
paper thing, not the right thing." That's not the intent of documentation. Paperwork should always work for us, not against us. In
healthcare, paper that isn't alive is worthless. There's a form for
everything it seems, but don't let your patient get the impression
you are primarily a paper pusher. Spend a few moments just talking with the patient before you put pen to paper.

DETERMINE THE PATIENT'S POINT OF CURIOSITY

"Starting with what the (patient) wants to know is a good
maxim to follow, even if that information is not the most important
for the patient to know to care for himself," advises Barbara

Gessner (1983, p. 593). Before adults will open their mind to learning, they must identify a need to know the information being presented. If a patient asks, "What's that thingamabob?" begin with what interests him or her and work in your own agenda. Don't try to make a square peg fit a round hole. Yet there are circumstances when the nurse must instruct patients about critical aspects of illness or treatment, rather than wait until they verbalize interest in learning. "My son, who has bipolar disorder, kept saying, 'I like it when I have extra energy and feel good,'" remembers his mother, a college professor. "But the nurse explained that he desperately needed to learn about the signs and symptoms of a manic phase. Otherwise, he could become exhausted or nutritionally depleted and get into very real trouble."

"I've found it helpful to close my educational sessions with this question: 'Is there anything you want to tell me that I haven't asked you?'" says a nurse practitioner. "Sometimes a patient will have nothing else to add, but it sure gives them a great feeling to be asked for input."

"When the nurse was teaching me about my diet, she asked me if I'd been having any abdominal pain," remembers a patient. "I'd just got through telling her a long story about how bad my stomach hurts when I eat spicy foods. I guess she wasn't paying attention." Some nurses have become more comfortable with paperwork than listening to patients. So often when we appear to be listening, we're just rehearsing in our minds what we're planning to say next or what we're going to write in the next line on a form. Listen to your patients closely enough, and they'll tell you what's wrong and how you can help them. Each patient is different, like no other one you have ever, or will ever, encounter.

BREAK IT DOWN INTO MANAGEABLE BITS

What's simple to us nurses is anything but simple to our patients and their families. Particularly when education is complex, tasks may need to be broken down into smaller, manageable doses to avoid overwhelming them. Reinforce information through repetition and paraphrasing.

Watch for yawning and fidgeting, which indicate a waning attention span. If a patient says, "That's fine for now, but I don't know how I'll ever remember it all," consider it a clue that additional information may be needed.

UTILIZE THE APPROPRIATE APPROACH

Sometimes we inadvertently select an improper technique for a particular patient or educational objective. "I thought videos would be an excellent resource for my patients who are illiterate," says an operating room nurse. "But then I learned that illiteracy is far more than the inability to read. They really need a staff member there to help them process the information, because their vocabulary may be extremely limited." Be flexible and change your strategies when necessary.

And don't overlook one of your best opportunities for teaching—silence. It's quite common to be uncomfortable with silence, but many nurses have learned that silence often speaks volumes about a patient's anxieties. If you don't always try to fill the void with empty chatter, you may well learn one of your patient's most heartfelt concerns.

PRAISE, PRAISE, PRAISE

My garden guide says that the most critical requirement of most plants is sunlight. Just as flowers grow in the direction of the sun, people, too, grow in the direction of positive reinforcement. When educating adults, remember they need specific, honest feedback as to how they are progressing. Catch your patients doing it right and praise them immediately (McGinnis, 1985). Applause! Applause! Praise, in fact, has been found to be a better motivator than a toy for youngsters.

If you do need to offer constructive criticism, ensure privacy and take timing into consideration. "Telling a patient his technique isn't quite up to snuff at the end of your shift isn't a good idea," observes a nurse on a cardiac care unit. "It may seem like an innocent comment to us, but patients with little to occupy their time may stew about it for hours."

In still another way, patient education resembles a garden. It's a work in progress. No one ever learns it all, including us. Offer praise at each point of the process.

RECOGNIZE THE PATIENT'S AREAS OF EXPERTISE

Everyone we meet is wiser than us in some way, and can teach us something. If we are open-minded, we'll learn valuable lessons from our patients we can pass on. Not only that, our customers will feel better about themselves and more satisfied with their care.

"When I was in the hospital," remembers a patient with gout, "they talked to me like I was a child. It was like, 'now I'm the mother and I know what's best.' That didn't go over well at all with me." How much better to demonstrate a sincere interest in the patients. Get them talking about themselves.

Bear in mind that even a patient who has not been employed outside the home has abundant life experiences which have served as invaluable lessons in setting priorities and learning organizational skills. Has that middle-aged homemaker been the president of the P.T.A.? Has your truck driver patient led a local Boy Scout troop? Find out, and you'll have a better perspective of how that individual learns and functions.

You know your desired outcome of patient education. Use the patient's experiences to help you reach that destination. Think of yourself as a road map, a tour guide. But let the patients drive their own bus. Our patients will model our behavior. That's why what we do and how we do it is so very, very important.

RECOGNIZE LIMITATIONS

Admittedly, there are those situations where you can't teach everything you've hoped for. This is frustrating for nurses who so often want to "fix" everything and have a tendency to take on others' problems they have little or no control over. It's important to assess motivation, which varies greatly from patient to patient. Internal motivation is always preferable to external motivation. When patients tell you they want to learn to change their dressing because gaining new skills gives them a feeling of personal satisfaction, you have a better teaching candidate than the one who wants to learn merely to impress his kids. If you listen closely enough, you'll discover what motivates an individual (McGinnis, 1985).

If the patient has barriers to learning, assess the family's or significant other's potential to reinforce and/or follow the educational plan. Referrals to outside agencies may be necessary to augment patient/family skills and resources, and should be initiated early on.

TAKE YOUR CUES FROM THE PATIENT

Before beginning any patient education, assess what else is happening in the patient's and family's life. "I cared for a lady who had undergone a total hip replacement," remembers a nurse, "and she was so resistant to her rehabilitation program. Then we found out that her father, who made his home with her, was in the end stage of ALS. To make matters worse, her husband had just been laid off from work. She just couldn't cope with the thought of getting better and having to go home."

Speaking of coping, it's also important to evaluate what phase in the coping process a patient is in before attempting patient education. If newly diagnosed tuberculosis patients are still in denial, chances are the best efforts at teaching them about their medication regimen won't reap lasting benefits. Acutely ill patients and those experiencing severe stress should be instructed in basic survival skills only until such situations have stabilized (Peragallo-Dittko, 1994).

AVOID MEDICAL-ESE

"My doctor speaks another language," complains a coal miner who was recently diagnosed with COPD. When patients aren't familiar with the jargon we routinely use, they quickly become baffled or intimidated, but may not ask questions for fear of humiliation (Christopher & Lajkowicz, 1993). A mother of a teenager with AIDS was overheard whispering to the checkout clerk at the grocery: "They put Debra on a protocol. What's a protocol?" When we use an unfamiliar term, it's best to follow it up with a word the patient is familiar with.

A husband of a woman with multiple sclerosis says: "The nurses asked me things they really should have asked Mary, but they said she was so stoic, they couldn't find out anything from her. Hearing herself described as 'stoic' just killed Mary's spirit."

The same goes for abbreviations. We nurses rattle off our lingo ... NPO ... NKA ... foley ... SOB.... We know what we mean, but to a patient these phrases may even have negative connotations. To complicate matters, every nursing and medical specialty has its own brand of jargon and abbreviations which creates additional distance.

A patient who spoke limited English was asked to give the lab a clean-catch urine specimen. When they analyzed it, however, it was water. As it turned out, the patient had merely dipped the cup into the toilet bowl, then urinated. Keep in mind that every culture and subculture (and even some families) have their own language which may seem foreign to outsiders, and may create barriers to following instructions or recommended treatment.

BE AWARE OF YOUR NON-VERBAL COMMUNICATION

A large amount of communication takes place on a level apart from the actual words we use. Smile. Make eye contact. Use appropriate touch and other non-verbal communication congruent with your spoken message.

Patients can sense when we're really not with them. Focus on more than just the words they are saying. Resist the urge to interrupt or to complete what the patient is trying to tell you, and you'll be less likely to jump to incorrect assumptions. Something as benign as glancing at your watch while waiting for a patient to complete a return demonstration can communicate a "let's get this over with" message and undermine an otherwise excellent patient education session. Failure to accept a treatment regimen is often related to miscommunication (Brown, Nelson, Bronkesh, & Wood, 1993).

USE THE NURSING PROCESS IN PATIENT EDUCATION

The four steps of the nursing process – assessment, planning, implementation, and evaluation – are the cornerstones of providing seamless continuity in patient education. Although assessment and planning begin at the initial encounter with the patient, they are ongoing processes that build throughout all contacts (inpatient and outpatient) with the healthcare system. When it comes to the implementation phase, remember the three basic tenets of public speaking: Tell them what you're going to tell them. Tell them. Then tell them what you've told them.

In evaluating the long-term effects of patient education, assess outcomes such as changes in attitude and behavior. Did the patient with coronary artery disease stop smoking as a result of your medical center's smoking cessation classes? Is the patient with COPD now using pursed-lip breathing techniques in appropriate situations?

These and other changes should be a part of the ongoing reassessment process on subsequent admissions and clinic or office appointments. And if a patient is readmitted with the same problem he or she was recently hospitalized with, that's a red flag that patient education may have been inadequate.

DON'T ASSUME THAT JUST BECAUSE YOU'VE TAUGHT A PATIENT, LEARNING HAS TAKEN PLACE

Often, in an effort to please us, patients won't ask any questions. Or they'll nod their heads like they understand everything perfectly. Sometimes they latch onto phrases. As one lady said, "I can repeat one of those big medical words and they'll think I'm smart, but I don't really understand all this radiation and chemo and when you do what."

A story is told about a nurse who thought she'd taught her newly diagnosed diabetic patient the ins and outs of insulin administration. But when the man was seen in the ER with a blood sugar of 380, he revealed he'd been injecting the orange, not himself, "just like they taught me in that class."

FOLLOW UP WITH PATIENTS TO EVALUATE THEIR RESPONSE TO EDUCATION

If you work in a same-day surgery or other outpatient department, it is important to call patients at home to assess their progress and answer any questions. When patients are still woozy from medication, they may not remember all you've told them. This is a valuable public relations effort, as well. Such a call can smooth rough edges or misunderstandings before they escalate to problems, identify developing complications, and may even ward off medical litigation.

Most importantly, a patient may be experiencing some difficulty, and you will provide an important link with the healthcare system. Giving a patient a calling card and telling them to "give you a ring if they have any questions" goes a long way toward engendering confidence. Remember, patient education plays a big part in their perceptions about the entire experience. Use customer input, too, in planning future educational programs.

THERE'S NO PLACE LIKE HOME

Patient education needs don't end once a patient leaves the hospital setting. Nowadays, patients are discharged sicker and quicker than ever before, and may sometimes feel like a houseguest who has all-too-rapidly worn out their welcome. As the impetus to control costs—and thereby release patients as soon as medically feasible to the community—continues, nurses need an arsenal of effective patient education techniques to prevent patients from slipping through the cracks of an increasingly complex healthcare system (Lowenstein & Hoff, 1994).

While the road to discharge planning may be paved with the most admirable of intentions, it is never a coincidence. To be effective, it requires the concerted efforts of many disciplines, coordinated by nursing. Patient/family education and discharge planning are interrelated (JCAHO, 1994). Yet nurses, however, are often unclear about the discharge planning process. Even case management and critical paths, which facilitate patient/family education at critical junctures and expedite movement through the healthcare system, are no guarantee that comprehensive discharge planning has taken place.

In one study, 61% of nurses stated they weren't involved in the interdisciplinary discharge planning efforts on their units, and 25% didn't feel that staff nurses as a whole participated in discharge planning (Lowenstein & Hoff, 1994). Nurses need to be oriented to, and participate in, discharge planning, and have an understanding of community resources, home health agencies, and transitional and intermediate care. "Identify needs for assistance and community referrals as early as possible," recommends a discharge planning coordinator who stresses that discharge planning should never begin on the day of discharge. "This includes their access to community resources as well as when and how to procure further treatment."

"Discharge planning can be as complicated as a house closing," chuckles a med-surg nurse. One easily remembered model for preparing a patient for discharge uses the acronym "HOME" (Liebman, 1993). Ask yourself:

How was the patient managing prior to admission?

Offer the services of discharge planning coordinators

Management problems at time of discharge

Educational and equipment needs

Also consider if the patient has another condition which hinders functional independence or self-care, such as arthritis, low vision or impaired sensory or cognitive function? (Tirk, 1992). Assess appropriate environmental concerns, too. If patients are being sent home on I.V. antibiotics, determine if they have electricity and a refrigerator. Does that patient who will need trach care have running water? How many steps must that new M.I. patient climb? Do they have transportation to emergency care should a problem develop?

While "home sweet home" is generally a lower cost healthcare setting, it isn't if patients become revolving door readmissions. In addition, patient/family satisfaction with the entire healthcare experience is significantly compromised.

Does the patient's family know how to obtain assistance if they need it (and know it's okay to ask for help)? "Many very capable family members think they can manage around-the-clock care until they really discover all that's involved or become overwhelmed with fatigue," says Sally, a unit manager who has worked diligently with her staff to bring discharge planning in compliance with JCAHO standards. "I used to get angry and think such families didn't want to be inconvenienced. But now I understand they need to know it's alright to say, 'I've had enough. I need a break.' After all, many are also trying to hold down full-time jobs."

And what about patients who, in our mobile society, have no family nearby? They must rely on the kindness of friends and neighbors for involvement in education and discharge planning. We shouldn't jump to conclusions about our patients, either. Diplomatically assess a patient's request for an early discharge. You may find the real reason lies in exhausted sick leave at work, not an indifference to health or your plan of care.

Be sure, too, that any discharge instructions given to the patient or family are provided to the community agency or individual responsible for the patient's continuing care (JCAHO, 1994). Forward a progress report, copy of the discharge summary, and any specific instructions to ensure that patient education continues to be reinforced by caregivers in the community setting (Tirk, 1992). This diminishes frustration and dissatisfaction for patients, families, and caregivers, as these days, complex treatments and equipment once reserved for I.C.U.s are used in the home setting (Carr, 1995).

When preparing patients for discharge, try to teach them using the same equipment and supplies they'll have at home. One home health nurse tells the story of a patient she followed post-hospital discharge. "They'd asked him to perform a return demonstration of his hand dressing using a little metal bowl from Central Supply, and he did great. He was instructed to do his dressing changes at 9 AM, 1 PM, 5 PM, and 9 PM. Yet when he returned for his check-up, his hand looked worse. His explanation? 'I couldn't do those dressing changes like you told me. At 9 AM, I'm driving to work. At 1 PM, I'm working. At 5 PM, I'm driving home. And I didn't do my 9 PM dressing because I didn't have one of those little metal bowls.'"

Any time you can incorporate discharge education into a patient's customary routine, you multiply your chances of success. A nurse who works in an orthopedic surgeon's office stresses the importance of helping patients adapt our techniques to their often vastly different home environments. "You might inquire, 'What's a normal routine for you at home? When do you get up in the morning? Alright, that's pill number one,'" she says. "Or, 'how would you do this dressing change in your bathroom at home?' You might find out they don't even have indoor plumbing."

If you're experiencing a niggling problem with discharge planning on your unit, why not snap a photo of it and then study it objectively (with regard to patient rights, of course)? One hospital photographed a patient going through all the phases of discharge. "Those pictures really captured the emotional side of the problem," remembers their discharge planning coordinator. "When we showed them at a medical center educational program, the staff commented that it was a wonder any of our patients ever got discharged. Did we ever see the need for change!" Today, the discharge process is now so hassle-free in some institutions that patients can actually complete it hotel style, right from their hospital room.

An important aspect of discharge planning is assessing outcomes and patient satisfaction. Consider telephoning patients, for instance, who undergo same-day surgery, or vulnerable patient populations with short lengths of stay, to evaluate progress and satisfaction with care and services. Most will be delighted to hear from a familiar caregiver, and you may well identify a needed intervention.

"When you send patients home, encourage them to feel free to call back if they have any questions or concerns. And if rapport is good and patients have had a positive hospital experience, they will call back," affirms a home health nurse. "It's quite another matter to adapt care to the home setting. Something as simple as having a business card with a telephone number to hang on the refrigerator goes a long way toward making a newly discharged patient feel secure." And when patients or family members do call back, return the call promptly.

The goal of discharge planning is to provide continued quality care and a smooth transition to the community setting while keeping customers satisfied. With the increased fiscal scrutiny of healthcare, we must, however, make certain we're not trading lower financial costs for a higher human toll (Carr, 1995).

DON'T SACRIFICE YOUR URGENT NEED FOR YOUR PATIENT'S IMPORTANT NEED

You've probably discovered that patient education doesn't always provide nurses with immediate gratification. "Sometimes with the limited feedback nurses receive from their peers, superiors, and customers, it's tempting to go for the immediate warm fuzzy," says a urology nurse.

But resist this temptation, even if you'll never know the full outcome of your efforts. We often have the mistaken notion that we have to make an earth-shattering difference in everything we do. But if we make a difference even for a moment, we make a difference forever. It's as educator Jesse Stuart aptly concluded: "I am firm in my belief that a teacher lives on and on through his students. Good teaching is forever and the teacher is immortal" (Stuart, 1993, Foreword).

References

Bader, M. M. (1988). Nursing care behaviors that predict patient satisfaction. *Journal of Quality Assurance, 2*(3), 11-17.

Brown, S. W., Nelson, A., Bronkesh, S. J., & Wood, S. D. (1993). *Patient satisfaction pays: Quality service for practice success.* Gaithersburg, MD: Aspen Publishers, Inc.

Carr, P. (1995). We can do that at home, but should we? *Home Healthcare Nurse, 13*(2), 69-70.

Christopher, M., & Lajkowicz, C. (1993, July). Patient teaching by the book. *RN,* 48-50.

Connor, T. (1992). *The soft sell.* Ann Arbor, MI: Training Associates, Int'l.

Cunningham, D. (1993, December). Improving your teaching skills. *Nursing 93, 24.*

DeVos, J. (1989). The patient with a brain dysfunction. In S. Lewis, R. D. Knowles–Granger, W. A. McDowell, R. J. Gregory, and R. L. Messner (Eds.), *Manual of psychosocial nursing interventions* (pp. 65-86). Philadelphia: W.B. Saunders, Co.

Gessner, B. A. (1983). Adult education: The cornerstone of patient education. *Nursing Clinics of North America, 24*(3), 589-595.

Harris, J. (1992). You don't know what to ask: A survey of the information needs and resources of hospital outpatients. *New England Medical Journal, 105,* 199-202.

Hemley, R. (1994). *Turning life into fiction.* Cincinnati, OH: Story Press.

Inguanzo, J. M., & Harju, M. (1985). What's the market for outpatient surgery? *Hospitals, 59,* 55-57.

JCAHO. (1994). *The Joint Commission 1995 comprehensive accreditation manual for hospitals.* Oakbrook Terrace, IL: Author.

Jones, I.H., (1983, Aug. 3). From a consumer's point of view. *Nursing Times,* 30-32.

Leino-Kilpi, H., & Vuorenheimo, J. (1993). Perioperative nursing care quality. *AORN Journal, 57*(5), 1061-1071.

Liebman, M. C. (1993). How do you facilitate continuity of care across health-care settings? *Oncology Nursing Forum, 20*(1), 116-118.

Lowenstein, A. J., & Hoff, P. S. (1994). *Journal of Nursing Administration, 24*(4), 45-50.

Lucas, M. D., Morris, C. M., & Alexander, J. W. (1988). Exercise of self-care agency and patient satisfaction with nursing care. *Nursing Administration Quarterly, 12*(3), 23-30.

Mason, J. L. (1993). *An enemy called average.* Tulsa, OK: Honor Books.

McGinnis, A. L. (1985). *Bringing out the best in people.* Minneapolis: Augsburg Publishing House.

Moore, N., & Komras, H. (1993). *Patient-focused healing.* San Francisco: Jossey-Bass Publishers.

Morgan, J. S., & Philp, J. R. (1985). *You can't manage alone.* Grand Rapids, MI: Zondervan Publishing House.

Padberg, R. M., & Padberg, L. F. (1990). Strengthening the effectiveness of patient education: Applied principles of adult education. *ONF, 17*(1), 65.

Parker, L. E., Wells, K. B., Buchanan, J. L., & Benjamin, B. (1994). Institutional and economic influences on quality of nursing documentation. *Health Care Management Review, 19*(4), 9-19.

Peragallo-Dittko, V. (1994). *A core curriculum for diabetes education* (2nd ed.). Chicago, IL: The Association of Diabetes Educators and the AADE Education and Research Foundation.

Pica-Furey, W. (1993). Ambulatory surgery—Hospital-based vs. freestanding. *AORN Journal, 57*(5), 1119-1127.

Press, I., Ganey, R. F., & Malone, M. P. (1991, Feb.). Satisfied patients can spell financial well-being. *Healthcare Financial Management,* 39-42.

Rankin, S. H., & Stallings, K. D. (1990). *Patient education: Issues, principles, practices* (2nd ed.). Philadelphia: J.B. Lippincott Co.

Rega, M. D. (1993). A model for patient education. *MED/SURG Nursing, 2*(6), 477-479, 495.

Spitzer, R. B. (1988). Meeting customer expectations. *Nursing Administration Quarterly, 12*(3), 31-39.

Stuart, J. (1993). *A penny's worth of character.* Ashland, KY: The Jesse Stuart Foundation.

Tirk, J. E. (1992, July). Determining discharge priorities. *Nursing 92,* 55.

Chapter 6

CREATING A HOSPITABLE AND HEALING ENVIRONMENT

I vividly remember my first stay in a bed-and-breakfast inn. As I turned into the driveway of the charming country home Friday evening after work, hospitality lights glowed in the windows and a "welcome" sign greeted me at the lamppost. The innkeepers, Dot and Dan, dashed out to the yard to say "hello" and escorted me inside out of the snow. Dan carried my luggage while Dot put the kettle on for a cup of herbal tea (my favorite—she'd asked what I liked to drink when I made my reservation). In my room were a bouquet of red tulips, a fragrant candle, and a stack of great magazines (she'd inquired about that, too). And on my down pillow was a heavenly chocolate bonbon.

With all that personalized service and attention to detail, I vowed never to spend another night in a run-of-the-mill establishment. They'd spoiled me rotten at a fraction of the price I would've spent at a chain hotel. Not only did I return there again to escape the pressures of the workaday world, I also recommended their services to family and countless friends.

Contrast my memorable experience with that of Mabel, a 74-year-old widow with arthritis and failing vision, who recently checked into her community hospital for kidney surgery. "My kids live out of town, and one of my church friends drove me to the hospital," she recalls. "In that maze of construction, it took forever to find a parking place. And when we finally struggled to the door with

147

my suitcases, we learned the check-in area had been moved to the back of the hospital. My knees were hurting, and my friend has heart problems. By the time they jerked us from one desk to another, we were worn out."

Mabel was "greeted" with mounds of forms to complete, shoved to her under a window by a clerk who, while gabbing on the phone to her daughter, couldn't locate Mabel's name on the admissions list. "Talk about feeling like there was no room at the inn," she says, throwing up her hands in disgust. "I was obviously a big bother, especially when I tried to ask a question. My friend joked that they should have posted a sign outside the hospital that said 'Prepare for Sudden Aggravation.'"

Will Mabel return to that facility if she has a choice in the matter? Will she recommend their "welcoming committee" to her friends and family? Probably not. The way she was treated didn't even come close to her expectations, much less exceed them.

In today's competitive world of healthcare, facilities that take hospitality seriously are the ones reaping repeat business. Hospitality is no longer an antiquated term that describes a visit to Grandma's house. It is an attitude of service, common courtesy, comfort, respect—in a word, caring. Or like my favorite innkeepers described it: "Hospitality is treating your family like company, and your company like family."

What the Experts Have to Say About Hospitality

Patients perceive their environments as either hostile or comforting based on their five senses. While the effect of the physical environment on health and healing is in need of research (Hutton & Richardson, 1995), unfamiliar surroundings are known to affect mood and thought processes, compounding fear and uncertainty (Walker, 1993).

Innovative hospitality in the medical setting is best achieved by consulting those with experience in both the healthcare and hospitality markets, say the editors of *Family Partnerships in Hospital Care,* a book on the forward thinking concept of cooperative care, where families are direct participants in the care of their members

(Grieco, McClure, Komiske, & Menard, 1994). While both markets follow similar procedures for receiving guests, the services provided and typical needs are quite different. Still, with more choices now available, healthcare customers are expecting more and more in the hospitality realm of care and service.

Healthcare organizations with a vision for the future are taking cues from those who provide red carpet service. Consider this advice from innkeepers at a bed and breakfast in Pennsylvania: "Don't peer from behind the curtain. Rush out there and greet them before they reach the porch. You know you have been preparing for hours, so why act so surprised when your guests arrive? Why make them ring the bell and then count to ten before opening the door and ushering them in?" (Greco, 1989, pp. 19-20).

While healthcare institutions haven't traditionally associated physical atmospherics with marketing, today's consumers are purchasing a complete product which encompasses the total hospital environment. Physical characteristics have been strongly correlated with overall patient satisfaction and perceptions of service quality (Hutton & Richardson, 1995). "To a patient, a commode that doesn't work says no one cares," observes a nursing assistant.

The Environmental Design Research Association, Inc. (Oklahoma City, Oklahoma) is an international, interdisciplinary organization whose mission is to enhance the art and science of environmental design research. The association seeks to better understand the impact of environment on patient recovery and worker productivity (Moore & Komras, 1993).

ROLL OUT THE WELCOME MAT

That's fine for inns, you might say, but what does that have to do with the efficient running of a hospital, doctor's office, or clinic? Think again. You've spent years in school and continuing education classes learning how to provide quality care to patients and their families. Your facility has invested intensive time in strategic planning, thousands—perhaps millions—of dollars in high-tech equipment, and considerable resources in meeting the standards of accreditation agencies. Shouldn't we, too, be anxious to serve our guests? Why would we want to keep our excellent skills and services a secret?

A hospitalized patient's room is their bedroom, their dining room, their bathroom, their living room (Walker, 1993). Interestingly, the very word "hospital" comes from the Latin word for "guest." With that in mind, I once asked an innkeeper how she accomplished the art of making her guest rooms so inviting. "Every few months, I spend the night in one of my rooms," she explained. "That's how I came to add the reading lamps. Our rooms were much too dark to curl up with a good book. And one night I almost fell going to the bathroom right in my own home. I installed night lights in all the guest quarters after that one," she chuckled.

"People often retreat to an inn at high stress points in their lives—an illness in the family, job problems, or to contemplate a major life decision," she added. "Comfort is a must, and unless you put yourself in your guests' 'shoes' once in awhile, you don't fully understand their needs."

You might be surprised to learn that patients who check into Presbyterian Hospital in Dallas are greeted at the door by a valet who knows them by name and is anticipating their arrival. With the admission process expedited, the valet escorts them to the nursing unit, where their room has already been prepared and their luggage has arrived ahead of them (American Health Consultants, 1994). It's true there's no place like home, but Mariott now has management contracts for one or more departments in over 1,000 healthcare facilities where their innovative "guest service concept" in the hotel industry is applied to the rapidly changing, depersonalized world of healthcare (Grieco et al., 1994).

Hospitals implementing patient-centered care are redesigning their environments to lessen stress and give patients a greater sense of control over their surroundings. This is consistent with the Joint Commission on Accreditation of Health Care Organizations (JCAHO, 1994) standard that healthcare organizations provide a safe and supportive environment for customers in a manner consistent with their mission and vision. Examples of innovations include enlarging rooms to accommodate family and other visitors; disguising the trappings of technology behind wall panels, an alley-like corridor, or inside a patient server built into an interior wall; and selecting wallcoverings, artwork, and lighting that is less institutional and more conducive to a positive mood and healing (Staff, 1993; Weisman & Hagland, 1994).

Don't forget the environment of healthcare staff who spend the majority of their waking hours in the workplace. William Arnold, III (1993), President of Centennial Medical Center in Nashville, Tennessee, noticed the housekeeping lounge was outfitted with dilapidated chairs with stuffing oozing from duct-taped wounds in the upholstery. Arnold, who employs over 2,000 associates, decided that quality improvement necessitated he consider their self-esteem as well as the patient's concerns. The very next morning he traded his executive furnishings for the housekeeping staff's castoffs.

The Joint Commission is concerned about environmental issues as well. Surveyors typically visit patient care areas to assess general appearance and infection control concerns as well as sensibility of the physical layout. Is clean linen, for instance, separate from soiled linen, and kept covered? Is the environment conducive to the diversity of your patient population?

THROUGH THE PATIENT'S EYES

It may not be feasible to spend a night at your workplace to determine how a patient might interpret the environment and service. But you can explore ways to make the impersonal world of healthcare as close to "home sweet home" as possible. For our guests are experiencing possibly the greatest vulnerability, loss of identity, and stress in their entire lives. Creating a warm, sensitive atmosphere is one way to bolster their self-esteem and confidence in the great care you provide.

The minute you walk in a business you can sense if quality and attentiveness to the customer's needs are a priority. Take a look at your surroundings as though you were seeing them for the first time. Ask yourself and your coworkers, "How would I like to wake up after surgery in this room or have a physical examination in this office?" Then make suggestions to the appropriate decision makers in your facility.

Or better still, ask your patients how the surroundings and service could be improved. This interchange doesn't have to take place during a formal satisfaction survey. Nurses are accustomed to doing several things at once. While giving a bed bath, you might ask, "Mrs. Hedgecock, did our new thermal blankets keep you warm last night?" If a sight-impaired patient tells you he "stumbled to the bathroom, feeling the furnishings as if they were Braille," take that comment seriously, especially if you hear several patients making similar observations. Keep in mind, in a healthcare organization, it's largely the nurse who creates the mood.

Yes, only our customers can really tell us how well we're doing. In our busy-ness (and with our eye focused on clinical issues), we may not see the obvious problem or solution. Interestingly, because nurses are the largest and most visible group of healthcare providers, patients often judge the quality of nursing care based on the entire organizational experience (Bader, 1988; Spitzer, 1988). For this very reason, in some hospitals, housekeeping, clerical, and other services are directly accountable to the nursing department, so that continuity of care and service are maximized.

It's essential that service and hospitality be viewed as an integral part of therapeutic intervention, stresses Leann Strasen (1988). For when these expectations are met, patients are less frustrated and respond better to medical treatment.

HOSPITALITY IS RARELY HAPPENSTANCE

We must make a concerted effort to create an atmosphere of hospitality because environmental comfort contributes to total physical and psychological comfort (Kirk, 1993). Part of serving our customers is customizing the environment for them. Still, we'll never achieve all the comforts of home, nor is that our appropriate focus. And no amount of pampering, amenities, decor, and smiles, of course, will ever compensate for incompetence and poor quality care. That would be like dining in a plush restaurant and learning that the kitchen was dirty. You don't want to return, regardless of how impressive the surroundings were.

Yet it is possible to practice the fine art of hospitality in any clinical setting. It's really a mindset. Offer a cot to a family member staying overnight, resisting the urge to grumble to a coworker, "What do they think this is, a 'Bed and Breakfast'?" Introduce yourself, and orient the patient to the strange, new hospital environment in a manner that says, "Welcome!"—not "Oh, no, not another admission." This is a splendid way to bolster consumer confidence in healthcare.

A nursing assistant shares this story: "We had an elderly patient in our nursing home whose wife lived way out in the country and didn't get to visit very often. One evening I fixed them both a cup of coffee. When I left the room, I heard him tell her with a chuckle, 'You know, Maw, I think the folks around here have kinda taken to us. You don't have to worry a thing about me being here.'"

To be sure, clinical excellence is never truly achieved without the service or hospitality component—part and parcel of putting the care back in healthcare. And it makes dollars and "sense." Simply put, patient satisfaction pays. Healthcare organizations that not only survive, but thrive, in the future will have a strong customer focus that motivates patients to sing the praises of the facility to others. "Take your care to the level where the customer will brag about you," says one hospital CEO. When an elderly gentleman asks, "Can I live here forever?" or a new father says, "No one ever checked my baby as thoroughly as you all did," consider that a great compliment and pass it along to the entire staff.

THE GOAL OF REPEAT BUSINESS

Sam Walton of Wal-Mart success recognized the value of customer loyalty when he said: "Making people want to come back.... That's where the profits come from ... people coming back over and over again." The Wal-Mart greeter is most assuredly no chance event. The guru of discount stores knew that customers form lasting impressions about an organization based on the first person they encounter. In fact, people make an average of 11 decisions based on their first seven seconds of contact with an individual or agency (Willingham, 1992).

But it's important to make each greeting sincere and not mechanical. The first time a doorman at a hotel tells you he's doing "better and better," it's refreshing and impressive. The twentieth time, when you hear him singing the same words to everyone, it loses its charm.

"A lick and a promise service attitude just doesn't cut it in healthcare any more," stresses a nursing instructor. The idea of 'satisfice—it's satisfactory and should suffice'—won't lure customers back, and does nothing to promote staff morale and pride. Many hospitals have competent and friendly volunteers meet and greet the public. One facility utilizes a warm, efficient volunteer to keep families of patients in the Operating Room and Post Anesthesia Care Unit abreast of any changes. Another assigns volunteers to the welcome desk where they not only inform visitors of a patient's room number, but also write it down on a pretty piece of note paper. Served up with a heart-generated smile, it sets the tone for the whole visit and is a wonderful public relations effort.

"When I went to the hospital for endoscopic surgery," remembers Sally, "a volunteer met me at the admissions area and escorted me to the Endoscopy Suite. What a relief! I didn't know my way around and I wasn't wearing my contacts. I was so anxious I would have surely gotten lost. Having someone accompany me really lessened my anxiety."

"This is just plain, common sense," you might correctly conclude. But unfortunately, the problem with common sense is that it's not common enough.

The impression you make on visitors will significantly impact future business. If a visitor is obviously lost, ask those five simple words, "How may I help you?" (some of the most welcome words in the English language). Or better still, offer to accompany them if you're headed in the same direction (Brown, Nelson, Bronkesh, & Wood, 1993). Did you ever notice the respectful, accommodating atmosphere of The American Red Cross? They pamper blood donors—their customers—with cookies and juice and all manner of comforting touches. That's in part due to the fact that donors come there on a voluntary basis.

If the atmosphere in your Emergency Room (E.R.) waiting area is typically chaotic, the problem should be addressed, not suppressed. If it can't be rectified at the unit level, consider organizing a continuous quality improvement (C.Q.I.) team to address the problem. But don't make things too complicated, nor overlook individuals inside or outside your department who may have insight and a valuable perspective. "In our E.R., family members were always bugging us for change for the vending machines," recalls Pete, a transport orderly. "One night they were coding a patient when a guy tugged at my sleeve and said, 'Got change for a dollar?' You wouldn't believe how simple the solution was. We arranged for a change machine to be installed in the vending areas, and the hassle factor dropped dramatically."

YOU NEVER GET A SECOND CHANCE AT A FIRST AND LASTING IMPRESSION

But how can you make a good first, and enduring, impression, especially when you're busy and short staffed? The answer is deceptively simple, and has its roots in the golden rule. Treat your customers as you'd like to be treated. A sincere smile and helpful attitude, eye contact and other positive body language, and an appreciation for cultural diversity and physical disability, all communicate volumes to a frightened patient while creating a warm, therapeutic environment (Brown et al., 1993).

If a patient is experiencing an unusually lengthy delay (one of the greatest sources of patient irritation), explain the reason, approximate waiting time (Hill, Bird, & Hopkins, 1992), and offer the option of rescheduling ("Mr. Smith, Dr. Johnson is going to be tied up with an emergency for about 30 more minutes. Would you prefer to wait or would you like to make another appointment?"). Giving customers a choice shows consideration and allows them to feel in control. Consider buffering that inconvenience with a warm beverage, especially if patients have gone out of their way to change their work or personal schedule to accommodate the appointment.

Offer a blanket to the young, single mother who's spending the night on Pediatrics with her sick toddler. We communicate caring by addressing the needs of the whole family. Remember, patients and their visitors think of you for their future healthcare needs if you leave them feeling good about you. As the Ritz-Carlton affirms, it's important to bid guests "a fond farewell" (Willingham, 1992, p. 98). For patients who are familiar with a particular hospital before admission are more likely not only to choose that hospital, but to be satisfied with their experience and recommend it to others in the future (Jensen, 1989).

Here are some other important considerations:

- **Noise Control**

    One of the most common sources of environmental irritation in healthcare facilities is noise, and it can even be a major factor in patient dissatisfaction with nursing care (Spitzer, 1988). "After my baby was born, I was exhausted," relates a first-time mom. "I would just get to sleep when the night nurse's shrill voice would pierce the corridor like a siren. Then the housekeeping crew would start mopping the halls. Couldn't they do that when patients weren't trying to rest"? Clanging dietary trays, a roommate's throbbing radio, paging systems, telephones ringing in the night, and beeping machines can grate on already frazzled nerves. We've all heard patients muse that "a hospital is no place to come and rest." Try to avoid using the patient intercom as a public address system. While some noise is unavoidable in an efficient hospital, carefully consider patient concerns to see if an opportunity for improvement can be negotiated.

    If a nerve-wracking noise can't be silenced, consider offering the patient a headset with some relaxing nature sounds or soft music. An extremely quiet environment can be just as distracting for a fearful, anxious patient. While some patients relish such quietude, others will benefit from a recording of soothing piano music or their grandchildren's voices.

• **Safety**

A part of any healthcare risk management program is the prevention of injury to customers (Grieco et al., 1994). Every patient is at some risk for potential injury due to just being away from home and the normal routine and environment. When making rounds, assess your patient's room with a global view to promote a secure, minimal-risk environment. Does it meet the needs of your elderly and disabled patients (Brown et al., 1993)? This is all part of developing a guest relations focus.

"When I was in Intensive Care, there was a terrible shortage of electric outlets," remembers one patient. "They plugged in my machines with extension cords, and that tangle of heavy orange cords was a safety hazard. They were always making comments about the equipment 'never working right.' How could I really feel confident about a place like that?"

Is your organization's smoking policy enforced? Is the traffic flow and lighting in clinical areas as efficient as possible? Do stairways have handrails? Are there cane, walker, and wheelchair accesses (Brown et al., 1993)? Instead of merely checking the patient's I.V. on piggyback rounds, look to see if there are trash cans, bedside commodes, or equipment that might pose a particular risk (especially in a small or already crowded room).

Don't underestimate the importance of calendars, clocks, bulletin boards, and other reality checks for your elderly, confused, or I.C.U. patients. Have you considered a bulletin board near the nurses' station with the photos and names of all unit staff members? A ventilator-dependent patient who was confined to I.C.U. for several months scribbled on a scratch pad: "I'm out of touch—I don't even know what day it is." "Don't feel bad," her visitor joked, "On the chalkboard in the nurses' station it says 'Today is January 26. Have a nice day.'" It was February 18.

Are patients' call lights within reach and do they know how to use them? Are the dietary tray and water where they can easily find them? Are needle boxes and metal baskets for gloves and masks within easy reach of nurses? (While this is primarily a staff safety concern, if it's not addressed, nurses will become frustrated, and this will adversely affect patient care.) Be mindful that safety—the very foundation of Maslow's hierarchy of needs—is a paramount basic concern of all people: patients, visitors, and staff.

- **Telephone Etiquette**

One of the most overlooked areas for creating a welcoming warmth on your unit is the manner in which the telephone is answered. That's often a customer's first point of contact with your organization. "Good morning—please hold" sends a confusing message at best.

"Myrna, the secretary on Orthopedics, smiles when she answers the phone," says an X-ray technician. "I can just feel her enthusiasm, and I love to call her unit because of it." Remember, other departments and healthcare agencies are our "customers" too, and the way we treat them trickles down to the patient and sets the atmosphere for working well with the entire healthcare team.

One nurse manager on a busy surgical floor makes it a habit to telephone her unit from home every week or so. If the phone rings off the hook (five rings is the acceptable standard for the unit), or she gets placed on the eternal hold button, she addresses the problem accordingly. It's a way of putting a mirror up to her unit to see things through the customer's eyes. It's said that a tiger who doesn't prowl is a potential rug. Management in today's competitive customer-oriented healthcare environment is part prowling.

Another important consideration is to keep personal calls conducted within earshot of customers to an absolute minimum. Patients and visitors may easily misinterpret a one-sided conversation held at the nurses' station, and this may undermine their confidence or respect in their caregivers.

One patient recalls: "I was sitting in my psychiatrist's office when I overheard his receptionist tell someone on the phone: 'He works us to death so he can live high on the hog and take cruises. Then he comes back and treats us terrible.' I never felt the same about my doctor after hearing that," she says. "How could I feel good about their care when the staff didn't even pretend to get along?" Employee perceptions often filter down to the customers they serve.

Another patient tells a story of standing in line to settle up her account at her orthopedic surgeon's office. "The phone was ringing off the hook," she says, "and each time the receptionist would hang up the receiver she'd babble about the patient she'd just spoken to. I know she was busy, but I decided to change surgeons because of that. Privacy and respect are very important to me."

Who's in charge of public relations in an organization? Anyone who answers the phone.

- **Be Innovative**

Encourage all staff to respond to customer concerns with a creative, personalized approach, going through the appropriate channels, of course. Did you know the average person works at less than 15% of their creative potential (Morgan & Philp, 1985)? Far too often nursing has taken the road less traveled. There is tremendous strength in the diversity of the interdisciplinary healthcare team. An ounce of different is worth a pound of same. The "way we've always done it" nursing unit or healthcare institution will simply not survive in the future. Part of continuous quality improvement is learning how to better collaborate with other departments to promote innovative approaches to care and service.

GOOD MANNERS ARE ALWAYS APPROPRIATE

Etiquette expert Emily Post once said, "Manners are a sensitive awareness of the feelings of others. If you have that awareness, you have good manners, no matter what fork you use."

Much of creating a therapeutic environment that nurtures body, mind, and spirit comes down to practicing good old-fashioned manners. When you're on a scheduled break, it's tempting to prop your feet up and let your hair down for a well-deserved few minutes. And it's important to take your scheduled breaks so that you can remain caring and hospitable to consumers.

Yet there are a few pitfalls to "letting your hair down." "The ICU. where I work is typically feast or famine," says a critical care nurse. "One night I only had one patient, and she was stable and trying to sleep. So I worked on a piece of stitchery to stay awake myself as I sat by her bedside. I didn't think anything about it until my husband asked me, 'If you were a family member, and you happened to walk in on a nurse needlepointing, would that make you wonder about the quality of nursing care?'"

"I was in the conference room sorting my treatment cards, scarfing down a sandwich," remembers a licensed practical nurse. "Would you believe a family member thought they saw me playing cards and reported me?" If you can't slip away from the patient care area, put a little preventive medicine on the situation and close the door. It's all too common for patients and visitors to spot nursing staff on break and draw the incorrect assumption that "all they do is sit around and drink coffee and gossip."

Nurses who smoke often find themselves in designated smoking areas with patients or visitors. In this setting, comments can be easily misinterpreted and the professional line between patient and caregiver and public image insidiously eroded. Take great caution to avoid "airing dirty laundry" in public. One family member remembers overhearing a disgruntled nurse complain: "Those E.R. patients are such pains." Little did the nurse know that his father was being evaluated at that very moment in the E.R.

It's all in the Details

Think, for a moment, of the difference in being served tea in a mug brewed from a tea bag, or sitting down to a silver tea service complete with scones and gourmet sandwiches. The end result is the same: a refreshing cup of tea. The experience, however, is quite different. While we can't host full-scale tea parties on our nursing units, we can be attentive to our version of "room service" details. For our patients, little things can and do mean a lot. Mother Teresa once said she didn't do great things, but rather small things with great love.

Findings from your patient satisfaction surveys will tell you what patients consistently complain about. For some, dissatisfaction may be related to temperature control; for others it may be the confusing layout of the facility or menu choices. Many of these concerns will need to be evaluated in an interdisciplinary forum. But for starters, ask your patients how they prefer to be addressed. If that 80-year-old former executive prefers to be called "Mr. Thomas," don't call him "John" or "Pops" or ever "the TURP in 339 B."

Just as important are the positive comments received on patient satisfaction surveys, or by word of mouth or personal letters. You may want to compose a scrapbook of heartwarming notes received from patients and families.

When you discover a valued service your customers remember, elevate it to a tradition of excellence in your work setting. "Our patients love the yellow 'Smile' stickers we give the kids (with a hug, of course) after they complete their school immunizations," says a health department nurse. "It's such a little thing, but we hear over and over again how those kids paste them on their lockers at school."

Don't worry if your department isn't exactly the Hilton; that's not appropriate anyhow. But do take heed from the experts in the lodging business who know that comfort, convenience, and caring are the three Cs of hospitality. These aspects of service are especially important for patients who, by virtue of illness, have lost some degree of control over their lives.

Just because healthcare has become big business that doesn't mean we should be so business-like we become detached. Invest in those small acts of kindness that give the heart a lift. The personal touch never goes out of style, and patients who are treated with sincere hospitality are much more forgiving should some misunderstanding occur.

TOUCH AS THERAPY

Nurses are recognizing the power of touch in creating a healing atmosphere. Studies have shown that touch is therapeutic to patients in terms of comfort, perceptions of caring, and relaxation (Talton, 1995). "Touch," says Bill Moyers (1993, p. 3), "is medicine's real professional secret." The more technological advances in modern healthcare, the more we need the appropriate use of touch—to balance high-tech with high-touch. Don't let technology get in the way of the therapeutic use of self—something only you can offer your patients.

"I'm . . . shocked and saddened by what I see nurses doing— and not doing," says Marianne Dekker Mattera (1994, p. 7). "I never see anyone touch the patient, hold a hand, sit down for a minute, eye level with the patient." Touch is important, but seek out permission to touch. Patients' body language will usually give you clues if they are uncomfortable.

Touch is therapeutic for both parties. I heard a story about a lady who gave her mother-in-law a back rub after she had surgery. While the woman had long voiced disdain for her son's wife, she suddenly began to open up to her, and they began to have a good, heart-to-heart talk. Have we nurses become strangers to touch? A new graduate nurse tells this story: "When I was fresh out of school and working the cardiac unit, I was giving a patient a back rub. An older nurse passed by the room and gasped, 'Don't scare me like that; I thought you were doing C.P.R. and hadn't called a code.'"

"Nurses are among the few professionals who have a license to touch," says a licensed massage therapist who is also a registered nurse. "And even patients who are resistant to touch will find it comforting during times of great stress. It's the most basic of all our senses . . . our first form of language. Touch is part of healing, and, 'puts the patient in the best position for nature to act upon them' to borrow a phrase from Florence Nightingale."

Is There a Reason for Your Rituals?

Human beings are amazingly comforted by rituals, especially during times of anxiety and great change. Yet with the advancement of technology, many basic nursing rituals have all but disappeared. Consider reinstituting the evening back rub ritual on your unit. You may be amazed at the enhanced patient satisfaction. And why not extend a gentle comforting shoulder massage to the weary primary caregiver of a hospice patient in the home or inpatient setting or, with their permission, to a coworker who is completing a double shift?

Now is also a great time to reevaluate rituals that have long lost their meaning and which may create barriers to seeing patients as individuals. "Since its early beginnings, the nursing profession has been embedded with rituals" (DeLuca, 1995, p. 139). But do all dressings have to be changed at 9 A.M.? Why not allow your patient who works nights and is used to falling asleep at 8 am some input into the plan of care? Do we really need to be so task oriented? Can visiting hours be more flexible to accommodate family members who work odd hours? After all, helping patients to "feel at home," through continuing their normal routine, has been shown to increase patients' confidence in nursing staff and help them cope with illness and disability (Kirk, 1993). Home is where people become their very best selves.

Never Let 'em See You Sweat

Today's patient care areas are more hectic than ever, but the more ordered and confident you can appear, the better your unit's overall public image will be. The fuss-budget staff member in a hurry but going nowhere does little to engender credibility. "If you look like you have it all together even when the unit is coming apart at the seams," says a psychiatric nurse, "patients are more apt to believe in you."

Hospitality is sincerely and simply honoring your guest, not thriving on chaos by complaining "you really have your hands full." It's not necessary to have flour all over your apron, so to speak, to convince your company you've been baking all day—especially in an environment that's already intense. The public is much more impressed with a healthcare team who functions efficiently and communicates calmly with each other.

CREATING A WARM, HOMELIKE ATMOSPHERE

When a friend drops by your home and is worried, what's your first gesture of kindness? If you're like most people, you offer them something to drink and find them a comfortable chair where they can relax. Those same hospitable touches go a long way toward telling an exasperated healthcare customer you sincerely care. Never underestimate the comfort of a cup of coffee or tea to a frustrated patient or family member.

"Nurses are seeking to discover the best ways to utilize the environment to optimize the overall healing effect," say Dossey, Keegan, Guzzetta, and Kolkmeier (1995, p. 290). The innovative staff on a pediatric oncology unit I once visited took the challenge of giving their work area a signature touch. The beautiful result was a more homey (although not overstimulating) atmosphere for patients admitted for sometimes terrifying and uncomfortable treatments. Previously unknown talents of various staff members surfaced. The nurses' station took on a serene outdoors look with silk plants and hand-crafted wreaths, and the halls were decorated with soothing, framed garden prints.

Now on each holiday, patients can look forward to creative decorations to commemorate the event. "We've learned to celebrate small moments around here, too," says a registered nurse who once thought working with young cancer patients would be a downer. "I believe having attractive surroundings with a touch of home . . . decorating an artificial tree with pictures of a patient's school football team . . . ordering them a birthday cake, for example, really helps our patients," she explains. "And we always encourage them to decorate their rooms with artwork and other personal touches such as family photos."

The Evelyn H. Lauder Breast Center, a branch of Memorial Sloan-Kettering in New York City, has displayed several hundred landscape photographs in its facility. Such decorative accents go a long way to lift a patient's spirits.

In one study, 80% of hospitals embarking on patient-centered care were remodeling existing space, while the remainder were beginning new construction (Staff, 1993). At the Griffin Hospital in Derby, Connecticut, patients in semiprivate rooms experience an enhanced sense of personal space thanks to an L-shaped layout with a bathroom in the center of the room. Rebuilt from the ground up with a focus on the institution's core value of patient-centered care, it is an outgrowth of its mission and vision, rather than the converse. The needs of family members were taken into account, too. A lounge with a full refrigerator, showers, and a covered balcony are but a few of the distinctive touches.

Interestingly, several of the hospital's senior managers have experienced healthcare crises themselves. Their personal input was critical to the project, as was the stipulation that architects, too, become educated on patient-centered care by spending time confined to a hospital bed (Weisman & Hagland, 1994).

"When I experienced nursing from the other side of the bed," remembers Sam, an intensive care nurse who was recently hospitalized, "I realized the importance of the small touches—letting me have a late-night snack because I'm used to working evenings . . . helping me arrange my get-well cards on my bulletin board. These are some of nursing's finest moments," he observes.

"My surgeon's office is so soft and comfortable," reports an elementary school teacher. "There are wing chairs and area rugs—you don't feel like you're in a doctor's office at all. I asked her about it and she told me, 'It's worth every penny I invested. When patients come here, they're scared. I wanted to create an ambience that would help them relax, because an anxious patient is a greater surgical risk.'"

In addition, patients heal and learn better in a tranquil, home-like atmosphere rather than a cold, antiseptic one. The environment, in fact, contributes to a patient's overall physical and psychological comfort (Kirk, 1993; Spitzer, 1988). In a study of postoperative patients, those with a view of trees as opposed to a brick wall experienced less pain and complications and a shorter hospital stay (Ulrich, 1984).

Families fare better, too, in a hospitable atmosphere, and the simplest measures speak volumes about the values of an institution. Is there a chair at the bedside for a family member who will be visiting for a long period of time? Looking at the environment through the patients' and family's eyes is well worth the effort. "You must imagine—truly feel—what it is like to be surrounded by technological paraphernalia and equipment with which you are completely unfamiliar," says Gordon (1994, p. 4). "You have to disregard your sense of control and succumb to what may seem a tyranny of schedules and routines that have little to do with your own rhythms and habits."

As Henri Nouwen observed: "The healer has to keep striving for . . . the space . . . in which healer and patient can reach out to each other as travelers sharing the same broken human condition" (O'Brien, 1989, p. 99). Showing patients and their families hospitality is always a journey, not a destination.

SPECIAL CARING TOUCHES

If a patient cared for on your unit dies, consider sending a sympathy card or note from your staff to the family. Unlike a phone call, a card or note can be read again and again, and is never an intrusion. This is especially appropriate if the individual was cared for by your staff for a considerable length of time. It's also an important form of closure for both family and caregivers.

Recalls the husband of a lady who died following a myocardial infarction: "The C.C.U. staff spent more time with my beloved wife during her last days than I did. They wrote me the sweetest note with some of the special things she had said at the end. I'll treasure it forever." One oncologist maintains a record of the dates of patient deaths and sends an "I'm thinking of you" sentiment on the anniversary of the loved one's passing.

An optometrist's office in my area mails annual birthday cards and "thank you" notes following each visit to communicate how much it appreciated the opportunity to provide its services. If such gestures are congruent with a sincere spirit of caring in the actual practice setting, the two go hand-in-glove to make customers feel valued.

CLEANLINESS

That old adage "Cleanliness is next to godliness" is never more apt than when it comes to the medical environment. Just as you wouldn't invite someone to dinner and not tidy up your house, you wouldn't "invite" the public to an unkempt healthcare facility. The general public is far more educated today than a couple of decades ago, and is knowledgeable and concerned about infection control and basic hygiene issues.

Visitors will judge the quality of your facility based on the appearance of public rest rooms, unpleasant odors, soiled linen tossed on the floor, a used syringe left on a bedside table, or the personal grooming of staff. The patient who has a roommate with pneumonia, for example, may be observing the technique of caregivers when you least expect it. "When my nurse didn't wash her hands between caring for me and another patient, I called her down for it," says Joe, who recently underwent surgery for peptic ulcer disease. "I'd seen a television program about those wicked 'knowscomal' [sic] infections and I didn't want to take something home to my wife and children."

Part of creating a trusting patient environment is attending to the atmospherics and the basics of good nursing care. Remember, while the public may not be equipped to judge the highly technological aspects of the care we provide, they do know clean, they know kind, and they know caring. Providing mouth care, shaving a total-care male patient, and brushing that bedridden elderly lady's hair is like putting a message on a public billboard that says, "We take pride in our work here." It's the best advertising in the world.

Take a Look Around

A hospital quality manager I know showed up unshaven for work one day during his first week on the job, dressed in a T-shirt and jeans. He brought along a stack of auto mechanic and comic books and parked himself in the clinic area "politely eavesdropping." When the day was over, he had far more information than he'd ever learned from the library or in his office—the aggravation of waiting, how old the coffee was, the friendliness and courtesy of the staff, how long the elevator had been out of order, how comfortable the chairs were. "I was more tired than if I'd 'worked' all day," he recalls, "and my back hurt." How's that for identifying with the customer?

While nearly all patients talk, dissatisfied ones talk even more. The typical unhappy customer will, in fact, share those details with 20 or more people (Press, Ganey, & Malone, 1991). From a patient's perspective, the environment and service are critical—the first things they observe (Hancock, 1991). And because dissatisfaction with healthcare is a much more emotionally charged issue than, say, an inferior car part, other people are much more inclined to listen up.

Sure, those innkeepers made it all look easy, but a considerable amount of planning went into that lodging experience. As a result, I went home determined to adopt some of their ideas. A healthcare facility that makes patients feel welcome, cared for, and good about themselves may well inspire them to make changes in their lives.

A century ago, Florence Nightingale wrote about the importance of a positive patient environment—ventilation, color, hygiene—in caring for the whole person (Skretkowicz, 1992). Today, patients who are pleased with their environment are generally happier with the entire hospitalization experience (Hurst, 1985). "The physical environment is to listening what the theater is to a play. No matter how intrinsically excellent the drama, it won't come across to the audience if the acoustics are bad, the props distracting, and the seats uncomfortable" (Morgan and Philp, 1985, p. 45).

Pay attention. Today's patients assess their healthcare environment with a practiced eye. If they are satisfied, they become trusting, loyal customers. If not, they may take their business elsewhere.

References

American Health Consultants. (1994). Valet, coordination are hallmarks of express admissions. *Hospital Benchmarks, 1*(1), 1.

Arnold, W. (1993). The leader's role in implementing quality improvement: Walking the talk. *QRB, 19*(3), 79-82.

Bader, M. M. (1988). Nursing care behaviors that predict patient satisfaction. *Journal of Nursing Quality Assurance, 12*(3), 11-17.

Brown, S. W., Nelson, A., Bronkesh, S. J., & Wood, S. D. (1993). *Patient satisfaction pays: Quality service for practice success.* Gaithersburg, MD: Aspen Publishers, Inc.

DeLuca, E. K. (1995). Reconsidering rituals: A vehicle for educational change. *The Journal of Continuing Education in Nursing, 26*(3), 139-144.

Dossey, B. M., Keegan, L., Guzzetta, C. E., & Kolkmeier, L. G. (1995). *Holistic nursing: A handbook for practice* (2nd ed.; p. 290). Gaithersburg, MD: Aspen Publishers, Inc.

Gordon, S. (1994, June). Inside the patient-driven system. *Critical Care Nurse* (supplement), 2-28.

Greco, G. (1989). *Secrets of entertaining from America's best innkeepers.* Chester, CT: The Globe Pequot Press.

Grieco, A. J., McClure, M. L., Komiske, B. K., & Menard, R. F. (Eds.). (1994). *Family partnership in hospital care: The cooperative concept.* New York: Springer Publishing Company, Inc.

Hancock, J. (1991). An assessment of patient satisfaction in hospitals. *AARN, 47*(10), 28-29.

Hill, J., Bird, H. A., & Hopkins, R. (1992). Survey of satisfaction with care in a rheumatology outpatient clinic. *Annals of the Rheumatic Diseases, 51,* 195-197.

Hurst, K. (1985). A question of satisfaction. *Nursing Mirror Research Supplement, 161*(12), 51-56.

Hutton, J. D., & Richardson, L. D. (1995). Healthscapes: The role of the facility and physical environment on consumer attitudes, satisfaction, quality assessments, and behaviors. *Health Care Management Review, 20*(2), 48-61.

JCAHO. (1994). *The Joint Commission 1995 comprehensive accreditation manual for hospitals. Volume I: Standards.* Oakbrook Terrace, IL: Author.

Jensen, J. (1989, July 28). Patients who chose their hospital are more satisfied. *Modern Health Care,* 66-68.

Kirk, K. (1993). Chronically ill patients' perceptions of nursing care. *Rehabilitation Nursing, 18*(2), 99-104.

Lumsdon, K. (1993, February). Form follows function. *Hospitals,* 23.

Mattera, M. D. (1994). Editor's memo: Where have all the flowers gone. *RN, 57*(4), 7.

Moore, N., & Komras, H. (1993). *Patient-focused healing.* San Francisco: Jossey-Bass Publishers.

Morgan, J. S., & Philp, J. R. (1985). *You can't manage alone.* Grand Rapids, MI: Zondervan Publishing House.

Moyers, B. (1993). *Healing and the mind.* New York: Doubleday.

O'Brien, M. E. (1989). *Anatomy of a nursing home.* Owings Mills, MD: National Health Publishing.

Press, I., Ganey, R. F., & Malone, M. P. (1991, Feb.). Satisfied patients can spell financial well-being. *Healthcare Financial Management,* 39-42.

Skretkowicz, V. (Ed.). (1992). *Florence Nightingale's notes on nursing: Revised with additions.* London: Scutari Press.

Spitzer, R. B. (1988). Meeting consumer expectations. *Nursing Administration Quarterly, 12*(3), 31-39.

Staff. (1993, February 5). Putting patients first. *Hospitals,* 14-26.

Strasen, L. (1988). Incorporating patient satisfaction standards into quality of care measures. *Journal of Nursing Administration, 18*(11), 5-6.

Talton, C. W. (1995, February). Touch—of all kinds—is therapeutic. *RN,* 61-64.

Ulrich, R. S. (1984). View through a window may influence recovery from surgery. *Science, 224,* 420-421.

Walker, J. D. (1993). Enhancing physical comfort. In S. Edgman-Levitan, J. Daley, and T.L. Delbanco (Eds.), *Through the Patient's Eyes* (pp. 119-153). San Francisco: Jossey-Bass Publishers.

Weisman, E., & Hagland, M. (1994, November 20). Built in care. *Hospitals & Health Networks,* 54-60.

Willingham, R. (1992). *Hey I'm the customer.* Englewood Cliffs, NJ: Prentice Hall.

Chapter 7

HOW TO HANDLE A CUSTOMER COMPLAINT

At this table, no man can complain that he is at the head or foot, lower or higher than another. Every man is equal . . . The names of all knights who sit at the table will live forever.
— Tales of King Arthur (Hibbert, 1978, p. 47)

For today's customers, satisfaction is no longer a nicety—it's a necessity. When they have a beef about something they purchased, be it healthcare or the latest kitchen gadget, the media are at the ready, telling them how to get what they want. And if the problem isn't remedied to their complete satisfaction, they take their business down the road—even if they have to travel further and spend more money to do it.

Let's say a patient (we'll call her Martha) has a mammogram at your facility and is shuffled through the procedure by a robot-like technician, who shrugs off her questions as "nothing to worry about." When Martha tells her doctor about the incident, he sloughs it off by saying, "They're awfully busy there, you know. I've tried to talk with them about several other complaints I've heard, but nothing seems to change."

Two of Martha's sisters and her mother have been diagnosed with breast cancer. One of those sisters died last month, leaving a husband and three small children behind. Martha read in one of her women's magazines that women who haven't had children are at an even greater risk for developing breast cancer. She confides her fears and her mammogram experience to a lady she meets at a business meeting. "Forget those flimsy excuses," the lady tells her. "You should go where I get my mammograms. They really take time with you, and even follow up with a phone call to see if you have any unanswered questions."

What will Martha do?

If she's like most American consumers, Martha will change providers and spread the word about her frustrating encounter (Willingham, 1992). Yet if Martha's complaint had been effectively addressed, there's an 82–95% likelihood she would have returned again and again, possibly even more loyal than if the unpleasant incident had never occurred (Career-Track, 1989; Willingham, 1992). That's important information, because it costs approximately five times more to lure a new customer than it does to maintain an established one (Willingham, 1992).

Let me give you a personal example. About a year ago, I underwent an M.R.I. preoperatively to identify the extent of new tumor growth in my head. The technician and doctor had to stick me repeatedly to locate an I.V. site to inject the contrast media. I was frightened and exhausted from being confined to that machine for what seemed like hours. "Can you do the test without the dye?" I asked in exasperation.

The technician stopped everything and for a few moments my anxious gaze caught her piercing blue eyes. "I'm so sorry you have to go through all of this," she said. "But if we don't visualize the tumors, the success of your surgery will be compromised."

As a nurse, I knew all of that on a theoretical level, but I wasn't operating on a healthcare provider plane. I was just another scared patient. Later, with the I.V. line secured, the technician added in a sweet, sincere voice: "And to think, you're from my very favorite state—West Virginia. I love to go there and ski."

An hour or so later, when I rejoined my husband in the waiting area, I found him sipping a cup of coffee. "They told me they had a little trouble finding an I.V. site," he said. "But they've been wonderful and even brought me a couple of cups of coffee." We left there raving about how gracious they were.

My surgery was a great success, but even before I knew the final outcome, I did a surprising thing. My arms black and blue from their unsuccessful I.V. attempts, I found myself at my computer, writing a letter of praise to the hospital administrator. Because they'd met us on a human level, I'd become a much more loyal customer than ever before—even when things had gone right.

WHERE ARE PATIENTS MOST SATISFIED?

When it comes to satisfying customers, not all healthcare organizations are created equal. Larger hospitals, as well as those located in bigger cities, those serving a large Medicare population, and those with medical school affiliation, are agencies which typically receive lower patient satisfaction scores (Press, Ganey, & Malone, 1991). "We should focus on providing teaching in a patient care environment, rather than patient care in a teaching environment," emphasizes a cardiologist.

But Press et al. (1991) contend the difference between service and technical components of healthcare may be an artificial one. The bottom line is that healthcare is delivered *to* people *by* people. Service is the means by which technical care is provided.

Dennis S. O'Leary, M.D., President of the Joint Commission on Accreditation of Healthcare Organizations (JCAHO), says: "In today's fast-paced healthcare environment, even a 'quality' product cannot afford to be complacent. Today, being good is not enough: getting better is becoming a way of life" (O'Leary, 1993, p. 211).

Some healthcare employees may fail to see the need for change, however. "We've always done it this way, and it's worked for us," they contend. "But chances are your closest competitor doesn't share that same 'status quo' philosophy," says Cox (1994).

LEGAL IMPLICATIONS

An attention-getting dimension of patient satisfaction which escalates healthcare costs, cynicism and detachment of providers, and erodes trust in the healthcare system at large, is the issue of litigation. Reasons for litigation include: perceived lack of concern or caring; discounting of consumer concerns; fragmentation; failure to understand or insensitivity to the patient's/family's perspective; breach of confidentiality; poor communication between providers, patients, and families; and adversarial contention between staff and patients (Calfee, 1991; Tanebaum & Berman, 1993; Beckman, Markakis, Suchman, & Frankel, 1994; Rubsamen, 1995).

Without question, more nurses are facing litigation these days. While some cases are due to errors in assessment, planning, or intervention, errors—even monumental ones—don't always lead to a lawsuit.

Interestingly, three fourths of all malpractice suits are related to patients' feelings about the care experience rather than actual injury (Scott, 1993). Poor communication has been implicated as a cause for otherwise avoidable malpractice suits. Again, that's because patients judge competence and service largely on a provider's communication skills (Brown, Nelson, Bronkesh, & Wood, 1993). It may be difficult to believe, but technical competence is often equated with a nurse's friendliness (Press, Ganey, & Malone, 1991). If a nurse encounters difficulty when inserting a nasogastric tube, for example, the patient and/or family will likely take it in stride if she is warm, sensitive, caring, and explains the reasons for the difficulty.

The best return on a healthcare agency's budget is to invest in teaching staff how to improve their interpersonal skills with the public (Press et al., 1991). Friedman (1986) brings home the important point that healthcare consumerism boils down to the *perceived* quality of care. While they can't differentiate whether the technical care received is an A, B, or C, they *do* know when it's an F.

Barbara F. Calfee, JD (1991), offers this advice for nurses in preventing litigation through sensitive communication:

1. Treat every person with sincere concern.

2. Don't address patients in a condescending manner.

3. Don't talk to others as if the patient isn't there.

4. Don't promise what you can't deliver.

5. Avoid improvising information when you don't have the answer, just to look impressive.

6. Don't complain with other coworkers or discuss poor staffing conditions.

7. Don't avoid contact with a difficult patient.

8. Always respond professionally.

The best predictor of whether a patient is likely to bring suit? The quality of the physician-patient relationship (Tanenbaum & Berman, 1993). Not only that, it can even enhance a patient's chances of a good recovery (Moyers, 1993). "I've noticed even in real calamities, people often don't file suit if they liked the doctor," says a risk manager. A man once said to me, "Doctors are human, too. I know mine made a mistake, but he didn't neglect me. His heart was in the right place and I can accept that."

Unresolved complaints often lead to legal action. Yet patients who are dealt with on a personalized level and have the sense that their complaint is being carefully evaluated are far less likely to file suit (Tanenbaum & Berman, 1993).

Every Complaint Is an Opportunity for Improvement

As strange as it may seem, you should try to make complaints your friend. "Mistakes show us where we need to learn. . . . When we make a mistake, it's a golden arrow saying, 'Study this if you want success'" (McWilliams & McWilliams, 1993, p. 411). Admittedly, being fair to the patient who is complaining while maintaining fairness to the organization is a delicate balance to achieve.

Is there an opportunity for improvement hidden in this somewhat annoying complaint? Instead of complaining to your peers that a chronic complainer has "elevated whining to a fine art," stretch your thinking to see the problem behind the problem.

Within an organization, complaints from internal customers (fellow nurses, doctors, other departments, etc.) and external customers (patients, families, visitors, vendors, insurance companies, etc.) are all in a day's work. But don't minimize them. As one patient remarks, "They don't take me seriously. They sidestep my problem like you'd walk around a bum on the sidewalk." Look for the lesson in each complaint and move forward.

When it comes to healthcare, most patients and families feel helpless and powerless. "What's the use of complaining?" they sometimes ask. "It won't do any good. They just tell you what they think you want to hear, if you can find someone who will give you the time of day."

Always look for a way to redirect a complaint into something positive. If a patient says, "This place is just like the bank. They're open when it's convenient for them, not their customers," maybe you really do need to take a look at the issue of access to care.

The JCAHO (1994) states that a mechanism which provides for resolution of complaints should be in place. Have a clear-cut system in your department for how customer complaints will be handled. If there's a policy or procedure, all staff should have access to this information. The last thing you want is a complaining customer complaining about the complaint process.

Most organizations have customer service standards in place. These should be posted in a public area or printed in a patient brochure, so customers know what to expect. If you are working toward a maximum 30-minute waiting time in your clinic, be up front and admit that this is your goal, not your current standard.

THE PROBLEM BEHIND THE PROBLEM

Let's say several patients tell you they are unhappy with the care they received in August on the Surgical Unit. You know that in August new medical and nursing students come on board, and that adds to the confusion. "That's probably it," you assume, and tell yourself that if customers are still complaining in October you'll look into it further. "Our patients have always bragged about our unit in the past," you reassure your coworkers. But that may not be the root cause at all.

It's sometimes helpful to take a look at lessons from the business world. The restaurant chain TGI Friday's was also once lured by past success. When their first seven restaurants opened their doors to the public in 1975, customers were lined up outside. Then sales plummeted 50%. When management looked into it, though, they discovered a myriad of irritations: crooked signs, waiters who were less than friendly, unkempt rest rooms. Their goal of being known in the business as a casual eatery had crossed over the line to sloppiness. Once those details were attended to, sales recovered. But that insight didn't come overnight. Every manager of every restaurant was charged with sitting in each seat of that restaurant at least once a month. Seeing things from the customer's point of view shed a whole new light on the problem (Whiteley, 1991).

Part of being detail driven is taking a good hard look at restrictive rituals and traditions in your organization that may, in fact, represent problem areas. "Tradition is important, but the voices of tradition can, in your head, become other people's voices that you're using instead of your own" (Rich, 1993). Ask yourself, "What didn't work for us in the past?" Resist the urge to be like the nurse who commented, "They don't pay us to think here." Maybe it's time to make some positive changes, and maybe those changes can begin with you. "Everyone's looking for ways to cut back," says an HMO administrator. "What we need are employees who are able to rethink the past, because many past practices have led to customer dissatisfaction."

AN OUNCE OF PREVENTION

Be proactive. Inform your patients of their rights as well as your complaints procedure when they seek care in your organization. Assure them that any complaints will be handled respectfully, confidentially, and in a timely manner (Staff, 1992).

"Always deal with complaints before they're made," advises Timothy Firnstahl, Chief Executive, Satisfaction Guaranteed Eateries (Whiteley, 1991, p. 1). Be proactive enough to identify your customers' needs before they actually materialize.

KNOW YOUR DEPARTMENT

Ideally, customers shouldn't be telling us anything we didn't already know about our product or service (Rosenbluth & Peters, 1992). What is the general mood in your department? Are your customers happy? If you were a patient there, would you be content with the care and the attitude of the staff? Encourage staff to ask themselves, "What does our behavior look like to a worried patient or loved one?"

Be leery of pat answers which can seem trivial to your customers. Rather, really get to know your patient population and their point of view. "They told me my husband was getting the best of care," remembers a lady who was disturbed over her spouse's prolonged surgical recovery. "They didn't even know my name. It really minimized all I was going through. I needed specifics, not band-aids."

RESPECT, RESPECT, RESPECT

According to Tanenbaum and Berman (1993), the failure to communicate respect is at the root of many complaints that escalate into legal action. Yet it's next to impossible for a person to remain angry with you when you're relating to them as an individual with worth; in other words, showing them respect (Scott, 1991).

Anything that violates patient trust sets the practitioner up for potential problems, whether it be communication breakdown, perceived rudeness, or unintentional breach of confidentiality. In matters of trust, never sacrifice the urgent for the important. The goal is long-term trust—a lasting relationship with the customer. In addition, if patients trust you, they're more likely to follow their prescribed treatment regimen and to perceive their treatment as superior (Press et al., 1991).

People are usually very reasonable when treated with respect. Try to handle the complaint immediately. "Irritation is directly proportionate to waiting time," contends one administrator. Remain professional and polite, and speak in a calm, controlled voice. Use open-ended questions to encourage the person to ventilate his or her feelings: "What happened to make you feel that way?" you might ask. Show empathy with reassuring comments like, "That must have been very difficult for you." And try to identify areas of common agreement between you and the dissatisfied customer. Such communication techniques will demonstrate that you are indeed approachable, and serve as a foundation for effective problem resolution. The "proper" words will come when you are speaking from your heart.

Why Don't All Dissatisfied Customers Complain?

Whiteley (1991) cites three primary reasons why customer don't always complain:

1. *They think it won't do any good.* Who wants to take on City Hall? It's no small task to find someone in a big healthcare agency who really has any authority to help you. "Sure, you might get a sympathetic nod from a receptionist," says Sarah, "but the people who can correct a problem are all dressed in suits in carpeted offices behind closed doors."

2. *Complaining isn't easy.* Complaining takes time, and time is people's most important resource. You have to find out who is in charge, when they might be in, then write a letter or make a phone call. That's a lot of work, and most people who threaten to do it won't really go through with it. That's why patient satisfaction surveys are absolutely essential. We must make sure that people have an opportunity to express a problem in the most expedient and confidential way possible. Cutting through red tape is one way to communicate that we take caring seriously. Patients shouldn't have to go through layers of bureaucracy to have a problem addressed.

3. *People aren't usually comfortable with complaining.* "I like to think the best of people. We all make mistakes, you know," says Erma Smith, who was inadvertently

given another Mrs. Smith's heart pills three evenings in a row. "Fortunately, I finally realized they weren't mine, and there wasn't any harm done." Yet while Erma didn't suffer physical injury, there is a problem on the unit where she was a patient.

Erma was reluctant to get anybody in trouble—"those nurses are so sweet and have so much to do," or to be labeled as a complainer. But what happens when Erma tells her blind sister about the episode, and she reminds Erma that if she couldn't see, she might now be dead? Remember, a passive, non-complaining customer may well be voicing dissatisfaction to your current or potential customers. That's why it's essential to keep an ear to the ground for dissatisfaction in your organization.

Patients in such situations will often switch providers before confronting an issue. But interestingly, while many individuals are reticent to confront a provider ("They'll have it in for me"), they will complete a satisfaction survey (Scott, 1993). That's why we must ask our patients to tell us how we're doing. Keep in mind, too, that evaluation is the final phase in the nursing process.

LOOK AT COMPLAINTS FROM ALL SIDES

In the past, a customer complaint would have typically been addressed to the president or CEO and gone through many layers of an organization before resolution. Now, they are often channeled directly to the nurse manager who is accountable and is given the authority for responding to the problem. This empowerment of staff enhances job satisfaction and morale, hastens customer contact from unit managers and responsiveness to customers, and lessens staff finger-pointing. When such a transfer of power is implemented, front-line caregivers (who deal with the fallout of customer complaints) have a more sincere interest and greater investment in making things work, because they witness results (Lewis, 1993). In this framework of trust, it is the *patient* who is at the top of the hierarchy, and this communicates volumes about customer care (Gordon, 1994).

Is it the first complaint this individual has registered? While every complaint should, of course, be taken seriously, a complaint generally represents only one person's opinion at one point in time. Use a common-sense approach and resist the urge to major on the minor. Know where to focus your intense efforts and when to smooth the rough edges of a simple irritation. "If it's not neuro-surgery, you may not need to be so precise," muses one nurse. But if you've heard a similar complaint from several customers, this puts an entirely different light on the matter.

FOLLOW UP ON COMPLAINTS

"I made a return to a mail order company," says Jenni, a nurse, "and they called me a few weeks later to see how the return process went for me. Had my VISA been credited? Was I treated courteous-ly? Would I consider buying from them again? I was really impressed, and have made it a habit to follow up like that with my patients who verbalize even the smallest complaint about their care. It's one way to lessen the fragmentation of healthcare . . . you lose so many of the benefits you've worked so hard to achieve if you don't follow up."

"When I purchased caller ID for my parents who are getting up in years," remembers Mary, a nurse, "the telephone company mixed up my order. '"Will I be charged for the time they didn't have ser-vice?' I asked irately. 'Of course not,' they reassured me. 'It was our mistake and I'm just sorry for all the inconvenience it caused you.' I knew they were on my side, and it changed my whole attitude."

Ask customers for input to identify a mutually acceptable solu-tion. Then follow up to determine if the patient is satisfied with the steps taken to resolve a problem, and use that data to prevent future incidents. And don't hesitate to tell patients that's what you're doing. This really sets you apart.

Never assume the problem will simply go away. If an individual has taken the time to register a complaint, it's significant. A study from Travelers Insurance, in fact, indicated that getting people to complain may actually be good for business. Just 9% of non-complainers who had experienced a problem involving $100 or more would do business with them in the future. But an astounding 86% of the complainers whose problem were resolved to their satisfaction indicated they would do business in the future (Whiteley, 1991).

Suppose a family member comes to you and says, "That doctor got my Mother all riled up. First he hit her with the news her cancer was back, and then he asked us if she was depressed. They can have that psychology garbage. If he can't do better than that, we want another doctor." The two of you come to an agreement that you will communicate the concerns to the physician on morning rounds. If you promise you will get back with them by 11:00 AM, follow through on your word. This builds loyalty and reinforces the fact that they have at least some degree of control in the frightening world of healthcare.

HOLD THE ANGER, PLEASE

Always keep in mind, you're in charge of how you respond to a patient complaint. But choose your words with care, avoiding trite comments like, "That could have never happened here. Our nurses always answer call lights promptly." Remember, it's better in the long run for a dissatisfied patient to express rather than repress, because eventually repression may lead to deep-seated dissatisfaction and even aggressive behavior.

If you feel you are under attack, try to use words like "help" and "care," and phrases like "I'll look into it right away." Better to acknowledge a patient's right to complain than to minimize the concern or try to silence a blistering comment. Patients see and hear things on a much different level than caregivers do. Use words that will convince them you're in their corner. For even the most angry patients will usually respond to a sincere interest in them.

An Attitude of Accountability

"This place is all talk and no do," complained a patient who had recently changed HMOs. "I decided I wasn't going to waste my breath again. Now this is the clincher. The last time I told them about a problem, they said, 'Well you just can't please some people.' Guess they'd met their standard of quality."

Even if you aren't the individual targeted in the complaint, if it's brought to your attention, it's yours for the time being. At Ritz Carlton hotels, the employee who first recognizes the complaint, owns the complaint. Staff are taught to do everything to avoid losing a guest (Brown et al., 1993).

Don't push the panic button, and resist the compelling urge to blame someone else. Assure the person that you want to get everything out in the open, get to the bottom of the problem, and arrive at a solution. Develop the attitude that you're working with patients with problems, not problem patients.

But in being accountable, don't unnecessarily berate yourself. If you make a mistake or behave inappropriately in a particular situation, take a second to reassess the situation and then another second to remind yourself, lovingly, that that doesn't make you a bad person. You can learn from the incident and become an even better nurse (and mentor to new nurses) because of it.

The Power of Perceptions

In the area of patient satisfaction, perceptions are everything. It's a common misconception that patients are most impressed with the latest in equipment and technical acumen. Nursing and medical care are so much more than this in our customers' eyes. And, surprisingly, new and improved is not necessarily better.

Many mysteries surround healthcare, and wherever there is mystery there is an opportunity for confusion. Maybe a patient read a nursing note on the chart and misinterpreted it. Take time to educate your customers about your business—healthcare.

Ron Willingham (1992), who is well-known for his seminars on customer satisfaction, often works with healthcare staff to help them articulate their mission statement. But he takes that exercise a step further and asks them to develop an exit statement. This is accomplished by visualizing an impartial person standing outside the organization querying each customer who leaves: "How would you describe the treatment experience you've just had?" Participants write desired customer responses on an index card. Talk about a moment of truth.

If you want customers to perceive and remember their care in a certain way, you can facilitate that response by interacting with them in that manner. How would your patients respond if someone posed the question, "How's the nursing care in that place?" "If we argue in front of a patient," says an office manager, "you forget it in 5 minutes, but the patient remembers it each time they come back to our office. They have so little to occupy their time while they're waiting to see us, that behavior like that looms large in their minds."

THE EFFECT OF MEMORY ON CUSTOMER COMPLAINTS

While it's true that more distant memories are particularly selective, even short-term memories can be highly selective ("faction"—part fact, part fiction), even though this may be unintentional. What this means when it comes to dealing with patient complaints is that all memories may be somewhat distorted. The longer the time lapse before the problem is discussed, the greater the chance for distortion.

Worse still is when the patient has discussed the event with a number of people who may have added their own perceptions and opinions: "the same thing happened to my mother" . . . "they let my neighbor die over there. After his surgery, no one even answered his call bell" . . . "I told you, Mother, we should never have gone to this slaughterhouse."

Certain disease processes, as well as psychological distress, also impact recollections. If you ask patients admitted with an acute depression about their childhood memories, for instance, you'll get a very different account 3 weeks later, after they have had a therapeutic response to antidepressant therapy.

Complaints registered within three days (and the sooner the better) have the least likelihood of embellishment. When patients decide to pay the past a visit, matters get complicated (Hagan, 1990). As Diane Sawyer once said: "I'm always fascinated by the way memory diffuses fact." Keep in mind that what people remember passes through their "need filter," another example that all behavior has its roots in need.

DON'T DISCOUNT INTUITION

Ever just "know" something you couldn't really base in fact? That's intuition, or a nurse's sixth sense. Trust it. It's based on past experiences, everything you've ever read, and a host of other sources. Intuition is a direct connection with your inner self and shouldn't be silenced (Hagan, 1990). Intuition comes from the Latin word *intueri*, which means to know from within. Dr. Cathie Guzzetta (Dossey, Keegan, Guzzetta, & Kolkmeier, 1995), a nursing research consultant, observed: "Assessing the status of clients holistically involves evaluation of data not only from a rational, analytical, and verbal (or left brain) mode, but also from an intuitive, nonverbal (right brain) mode" (p. 164). While intuition has not in the past been accorded the respect it deserves from the scientific community, she stresses "intuition is a process by which we know more than we can explain . . ." (p. 164) and is an essential component of quality care.

Have you ever sensed that a patient or family member was dissatisfied, although they never actually said so? Many are reluctant to complain directly. One family member relates this experience: "My grandma was in the hospital with a fractured hip. Because I'm a nurse, they asked me to bathe her after I got off working the midnight shift in the E.R. She's such a private, dignified lady—I'd never even seen her in her underwear. I wanted to complain, and they had to know I was irritated and tired. But no one even broached the subject with me."

Because patients are limited in their abilities to assess technical aspects of their care, complaints will often focus on those aspects which they can measure: cleanliness, noise, insufficient instruction, friendliness of caregivers. Sometimes patient dissatisfaction is like a low-grade fever. It's there, and it's a problem, but it's so subtle you won't detect it unless you're specifically looking for it. Let your intuition help guide your professional practice.

FACT-FINDING AND RECORD KEEPING

Reviewing the patient's medical record and other pertinent documents is an important part of fact-finding. But your prime resource is always the individuals you are dealing with. Repeat what they tell you to make sure you've heard them correctly. People usually calm down when they realize you are making a concerted effort to hear what they're saying and understand what they want. Resist the urge, however, to answer with tired clichés like, "I know what you are going through." Instead, restate what you believe the person wants and outline options for problem resolution.

Maintain records of every complaint, not just for legal records, but also so you can refresh your own memory of the situation. Such records should always, of course, be kept under lock and key. Suppose a patient's daughter calls you about a complaint registered several days before on your medical unit. You can quickly refer to your notes and say, "Yes, I remember you, Mrs. Jenkins. On October 10th we discussed the problem with your father's pain medication. I've spoken with all the medication nurses and his physician and we've worked out a new system. He says his pain is now relieved. How do things seem to you now?" As a result of your organization and attention to detail, that person will likely have more confidence in you.

TAKE A TEAM APPROACH

Involve other members of the interdisciplinary team, as appropriate, but don't place blame. Many patient complaints cross interdisciplinary lines and present an opportunity to improve care for several departments. If you identify a consistent complaint, you might want to consider looking at it from a continuous quality improvement (CQI) perspective (see Chapter 3).

Just discussing the incident with a non-nurse can bring fresh insight, too. Recalls a unit manager: "I remember a situation where I was trying to explain what had happened with a patient to our social worker who, of course, didn't have a medical background. She knew the patient well, but had great difficulty understanding what I was trying to communicate. I broke it down into simpler terms for her, and it was only then that I understood a lot of the patient's confusion."

Sometimes nurses are a buffer for complaints involving other disciplines. Remembers a nurse: "A patient's wife came to me crying about an incident involving her husband, who had recently suffered a stroke. The patient was trying to tell one of the physical therapists in our office something, but his speech was slurred. According to the patient's wife, the therapist had slammed his fist on the desk and barked, 'You're not listening to me.' When I sat down to discuss it with her, she admitted, 'It wasn't really that bad. It's just that he's my husband, and he's all I've got.'"

Nurses are often the first line of defense for patient complaints. Be committed to resolving them as soon as possible, whether it is a perceived clinical issue or a dripping faucet. Alert the nurse in charge, the unit manager, and the nursing supervisor of any potential discord, as appropriate.

The only time you should allow yourself to be truly "caught in the middle" is when all parties are committed to a resolution of the problem and mutually respect you. A patient complaint can get disciplines working together for the betterment of patient care. Adversity can bring a unit or team together. Strive for a win-win situation.

THE PATIENT REPRESENTATIVE

If the complaint can't be resolved at the departmental level, and you work in an institution where there is a patient representative (sometimes called an ombudsman), this individual should be involved.

The patient representative collects, analyzes, and trends customer satisfaction data, and is an important part of an organization's risk management program. As advocates for customers, they help patients and families understand policies and procedures and their rights. Addressing complaints and issues that often cross interdisciplinary or departmental lines, they focus on problems, not problem people. Their access to top hospital administrators places them in a key, but neutral, position to cut through administrative red tape. Patient representatives work with quality improvement teams as well as individual staff, patients, and families to identify problems and negotiate solutions, thereby restoring the therapeutic link between customers and caregivers.

The patient representative should be an approachable facilitator, not an adversarial guard dog. He or she should base actions on sound data from satisfaction surveys and other sources of customer input, yet possess excellent intuitive and communication skills. Such an approach will protect patient rights, and help prevent and manage perceived or actual problems before they escalate in a manner that will increase the likelihood of litigation and/or negative publicity about the institution (Ziegenfuss & O'Rourke, 1995).

A critical care nurse recalls the time he cared for a patient in respiratory failure. "I tried to explain to his wife how we were being aggressive with his care to give him the best chance of getting through it. I really spent a lot of time with her, and thought she understood everything. She smiled and nodded at all the right times. Next thing I knew, she'd reported to hospital administration that I'd told her I was being 'abusive'." In such a complaint, a patient representative might investigate the situation with the staff and family, and if no evidence of abuse or neglect was identified, seek to clarify terminology with the patient's family. Follow-up interventions might include a staff conference on effective communication skills for anxious customers, without placing blame on any one provider for the misunderstanding.

A psychiatric nurse observes: "Sickness and hospitalization place you in a very vulnerable place, where every emotion is intensified and brought to the surface. It's not uncommon for a patient under stress to read things into an encounter. Communication is the biggest problem we face in any relationship. Nurses are far more likely to get into serious job conflicts because of interpersonal problems than actual competence issues." Become a partner with your patient representative, a most valuable resource person.

EMPLOYEE ISSUES

When looking beyond the obvious, take time to ascertain if this complaint represents a trend for an employee or an isolated event. If this is the tenth complaint on a single provider, you have a far different situation than if that individual is generally respected by staff, patients, and visitors.

When a question of professional misconduct, negligence, or patient abuse (verbal or physical) is identified, a formal board of investigation should be appointed. This process balances respect and dignity for both customer and staff rights. Even if the allegation is deemed unsubstantiated or invalid, it nevertheless presents an opportunity to reexamine standards of care, organizational policies and procedures, and communication patterns. If the allegation is deemed valid, appropriate disciplinary action must be taken in a timely manner.

Sometimes, however, we nurses tend to be extremely hard on our peers. An employee should always be considered innocent until proven guilty, for a false accusation can wound a nurse for life. Deal with the facts, move toward a resolution, and don't keep stirring the complaint pot. Maybe they were just having a bad day, although one manager in retailing asserts that "while employees do occasionally have a bad day, the customer should never know about it."

Problem solving with patients should involve a creative approach that examines all angles, not merely pigeonholing or applying a Band-Aid to the situation. For more happy endings, listen to your employees at all levels of organization. Some of the best ideas will come from unlikely people.

Share your success stories, too. Everyone loves happy endings, and healthcare workers don't always witness a lot of them. Pay as much attention to what you're doing right as to what needs to be improved. Are nursing staff who are customer-service oriented rewarded at your facility? They should be.

HONESTY IS THE BEST POLICY

There's a little joke in the field of entertainment: "The secret to success in show business is honesty. Now if you can fake that, you've got it made." When dealing with dissatisfied customers, sincerity is the most difficult thing to fake. People want to be dealt with honestly and to be taken seriously. If you don't know the answer, ask someone who does. And never give the patient any indication that you are trying to cover something up. If you've made a mistake, apologize simply and sincerely.

WHAT ELSE IS GOING ON WITH THE CUSTOMER?

In the heat of the moment at the "complaint counter" it's easy to forget that perceptions are altered under stress. There are few stressors like being ill or having a loved one who is ill. The patient who ticks off a whole laundry list of complaints may be trying to tell you about a much deeper need. Instead of whipping yourself or your coworkers with blame, remember, a patient's foul mood usually has little to do with you. We can't change others' reactions, but we can change how we will respond. It's been said that life is only 10% what happens to you, and 90% how you react to it. In a word, attitude.

Give trying situations some emotional air time. Jane, a night shift ICU nurse, remembers a patient complaint with vivid detail: "I'd left a sick child at home to come into work because we were so short-staffed. I poured everything I had into caring for a new patient with a head injury. And what did her husband do, but go to the Director of Nursing's office the next morning and complain that I had a snippy tongue! I felt like someone had stabbed me," she says, her shaky voice fading to a whisper. "I sat there and lost it, thinking of my little girl in her pink flannel gown I'd left at home with a sitter. I wouldn't have given his wife any better care if she had been my own mother." This complaint was likely related to the fear and loss of control the patient's husband was experiencing.

A patient who can't control matters of life and death will sometimes become compulsive in the restrictive hospital environment.

"I remember a patient who was scheduled for radical gynecological surgery," says a nurse. "A friend brought her a basket full of all kinds of niceties. After she left, I found the patient scrubbing the price tags off the gifts."

Sidney J. Harris once said: "It's surprising how many persons go through life without ever recognizing that their feelings toward other people are largely determined by their feelings toward themselves, and if you're not comfortable within yourself, you can't be comfortable with others." Can we second-guess what's going on in the intricate lives of our customers? No. While all concerns—real or imagined—should be addressed, don't overpersonalize customer interactions and lose heart.

LET THE CUSTOMER SAVE FACE

"I marched into the hospital administrator's office the other day and really showed myself because the food was cold," says a restaurant chef who was hospitalized for cardiac arrhythmias. "But about half way into the conversation, I realized these were very nice people who were trying to do a good job. The guy took notes and asked me about my work. I wanted to crawl under the table when they offered me a cup of coffee. But he let me ease out of my embarrassment. When I turned to leave, he introduced me to a member of his staff and said he'd be letting me know how one of my suggestions worked out."

People often back down on their threats if you interact with them person to person. "I've got a knot on my arm where the lab drew my blood, and I'm going straight to the newspaper," spouted an outpatient with leukemia. The best approach? Deal with the issue raised, and if you sense the patient is only blowing off steam and there is really no problem, give them an out. Many people who complain are embarrassed and astounded at their outbursts, but won't back down to save face unless you offer them the opportunity.

Initiate Appropriate Referrals

Sometimes a customer will complain about a bill, an insurance hassle, or other non-nursing issue to the nursing staff. If this happens, don't say, "That's not my department," but rather direct them to someone who can assist them. If possible, pick up the phone and initiate the referral, then follow up to make sure it was attended to. "But that's not real nursing," you might say. That's true. Yet if you leave your customer hanging, you'll leave them with an unfavorable impression of nursing as well. People tend to judge the organization as a whole.

Make the Disgruntled Customer a Loyal Customer

Some of the best advice I ever heard came from a unit manager who told me: "When you have a patient or family member who is very intense, it's likely one of two things will happen: if they're pleased with their care, they'll be your biggest ally. These are the people who write letters to the editor of the newspaper. On the other hand, if they are unhappy with their care, these are the people who will complain the loudest. Might as well make them your friend from the start." That's not to say you pay more attention to people with this personality characteristic, but it is prudent to be aware. And if you don't take the time to make things right and try to dream up an excuse, it will mar every future encounter for that individual.

End every interaction on a positive note, if possible. Ensure patients of the measures taken to prevent a recurrence of the problem. And if you make a change in your organization based on a customer frustration or complaint, consider letting them know their input led to better service for other customers.

EMPLOYEE EDUCATION

An organization's mission, vision and CQI activities should be introduced at a new employee orientation, and stressed at regular intervals through staff inservice education. An important component is the organization's philosophy of customer relations and rectifying problems (Dugar, 1995). New employees may have previously worked in institutions that had a departmental-based QI program with an entirely different philosophy of customer service and handling complaints. With CQI, it's not merely bedside caregivers for whom ownership and empowerment should assume new meaning. The entire hospital organizational structure must be changed as well (Lathrop, 1993).

Still, peer pressure to conform to negative stereotyping of patients who complain (especially chronic complainers) is very real in healthcare organizations. Staff meetings are a prime opportunity for additional informal inservice education where specific situations can be reviewed (for example, patient incident reports or content analysis of letters received from customers), and preventive strategies for future occurrences and organizational improvement discussed.

THE HIGH COST OF PATIENT DISSATISFACTION

Patient dissatisfaction carries a high emotional and fiscal price tag (Press et al., 1991). For a hospital with 5,000 annual discharges, the yearly cost of patient dissatisfaction with hospital services is estimated to be $750,000.00 (Steiber & Krowinski, 1990). Clearly, it's better from all perspectives to do the right thing and to do it right the first time. It costs considerable money to woo back a lost customer. Bending over backwards to please our patients is not an exercise in futility. People, after all, will get their healthcare somewhere.

Norman Vincent Peale once observed that whenever a small wrong is committed, some mysterious balance is disturbed, and that balance remains as such until that wrong is righted. Making wrongs right, small or large—that's what handling customer complaints is all about. Customer satisfaction principles are much the same regardless of the business setting. People are people. No, our customers are not always right. But, hopefully, they'll always be our customers.

References

Beckman, H. B., Markakis, K. M., Suchman, A. L., & Frankel, R. M. (1994). The doctor-patient relationship and malpractice: Lessons from plaintiff depositions. *Archives of Internal Medicine, 154,* 1365-70.

Brown, S. W., Nelson, A. M., Bronkesh, S. J., & Wood, S. D. (1993). *Patient satisfaction pays: Quality service for practice success.* Gaithersburg, MD: Aspen Publishers, Inc.

Calfee, B. E. (1991, December). Protecting yourself. *Nursing 91, 91,* 34-39.

Career-Track. (1989). *In search of excellence: The seminar.* Boulder, CO: Author.

Cox, D. (1994). *Leadership when the heat's on.* Tustin, CA: Seminar Handout.

Dugar, B. (1995). Implementing CQI on a budget: A small hospital's story. *Journal of Quality Improvement, 21*(2), 57-69.

Friedman, E. (1986, May/June). What do consumers really want? *Healthcare Forum,* 20.

Gordon, S. (1994, June). Inside the patient-driven system. *Critical Care Nurse* (supplement), 2-28.

Guzzetta, C. E. (1995). Holistic approach to the nursing process. In B.M. Dossey, L. Keegan, C.E. Guzzetta, and L.G. Kolkmeier (Eds.), *Holistic nursing: A handbook for practice* (2nd ed., pp. 155-193). Gaithersburg, MD: Aspen Publishers, Inc.

Hagan, K. L. (1990). *Internal affairs: A journalkeeping workbook for self-intimacy.* New York: Harper Collins Publishers.

Hibbert, P. (1978). *The search for King Arthur.* New York: Harper and Row.

JCAHO. (1994). *The Joint Commission 1995 comprehensive accreditation manual for hospitals. Volume I: Standards.* Oakbrook Terrace, IL: Author.

Lathrop, J. P. (1993). *Restructuring health care: The patient focused paradigm* (p. 98). San Francisco: Jossey-Bass, Inc.

Lewis, A. (1993). Too many managers: Major threat to CQI in hospitals. *QRB, 19*(3), 95-101.

McWilliams, J. R., & McWilliams, P. (1993). *The portable do it!* Los Angeles: Prelude Press.

Moyers, B. (1993). *Healing and the mind.* New York: Doubleday.

O'Leary, D. S. (1993). Foreword. *Journal of Quality Improvement, 19*(7), 211-212.

Press, I., Ganey, R. F., & Malone, M. P. (1991, Feb.). Satisfied patients can spell financial well-being. *Healthcare Financial Management,* 34-42.

Rich, A. (1993, Nov. 29). Interview. *Publishers Weekly.*

Rosenbluth, H. F., & Peters, D. M. (1992). *The customer comes second and other secrets of exceptional service.* New York: Quill (William Morrow & Co.).

Rubsamen, D. S. (1995, April 30). Three scenarios that spotlight the malpractice hazards pervading managed care. *Managed Care Report,* S1, S14-15.

Scott, D. (1991). *Customer satisfaction.* Menlo Park, CA: Crisp Publications, Inc.

Scott, L. (1993). *It's a dog's world.* Carlsbad, CA: CRM Films Leaders Guide.

Staff. (1992). Patient complaints: Guidance for nurses. *Nursing Standard, 7*(7), 29-30.

Steiber, S. R., & Krowinski, W. J. (1990). *Measuring and monitoring patient satisfaction.* American Hospital Publishing, Inc.

Tanenbaum, R., & Berman, M. (1993, April). Why even patients who like you will sue you for malpractice. *Physician's Management,* 85-97.

Whiteley, R. C. (1991). *The customer driven company: Moving from talk to action.* Reading, MA: Addison-Wesley Publishing Co.

Willingham, R. (1992). *Hey I'm the customer.* Englewood Cliffs, NJ: Prentice Hall.

Ziegenfuss, J. T., & O'Rourke, P. (1995). Ombudsmen, patient complaints, and total quality management: An examination of fit. *Journal of Quality Improvement, 21*(3), 133-142.

Chapter 8

MEASURING AND EVALUATING PATIENT SATISFACTION FINDINGS

Looking for the Lesson

Oh wad some power the giftie gie us. To see oursels as others see us!
— Robert Burns, *To a Louse* (1786), st. 8

To see ourselves as others see us. On a busy medical unit, a nursing assistant escorts to the front lobby a newly discharged patient who had been hospitalized for hypertensive crisis. As the patient is wheeled away in the company of a smiling wife, his primary nurse remarks: "Now there's a patient I feel good about. I had the time to do all the important things, like educate him about his meds and arrange a consultation with the dietitian for him and his wife."

But two weeks later, a scathing letter arrives in the Office of the Director detailing the staff's lack of sensitivity to his privacy. The medical and nursing staff were overwhelmingly satisfied with his clinical outcome. But the patient, it turned out, viewed things from a totally different vantage point. According to him, there was ample room for improvement. "Makes you wonder what the rest of them are thinking," a nurse remarked when the letter was later discussed in a staff meeting.

In a follow-up meeting, the nurse manager shared her philosophy of analyzing the content of complaint letters to recognize weaknesses and improve performance. "So often, I've noticed, we're not interacting with our patients until we have conflict with them," she said. "We're reactive instead of proactive. I value all of your input, and I'd like to hear your thoughts on how we could work together to change this. After all, you are the ones who really make healthcare work."

All too often managers have responded with a knee-jerk reaction or have applied a quick fix to problems identified in the area of customer satisfaction. But a partial application of continuous quality improvement (CQI) principles and methods simply isn't effective (Gelmon & Baker, 1995); CQI must be a management style and a pervasive organizational philosophy.

The Importance of Feedback

The Joint Commission on Accreditation of Healthcare Organizations (JCAHO, 1994, p. 33) states that organizations should collect data about patient needs and expectations, including the degree to which these needs and expectations have been met. Patient letters and satisfaction surveys are important indicators of quality as seen from the customer's perspective. In fact, the very survival of CQI necessitates that healthcare providers identify what really matters to internal and external customers. If not, CQI could well become "buried in the graveyard of past management fads, such as quality circles and management by objectives, that captured the fancy of healthcare managers but failed to become incorporated into ongoing management practices" (Shortell, 1995, p. 5).

Feedback helps an individual practitioner or institution improve future performance by examining past performance. Clients are vital sources of feedback to an institution. While they may have limited expertise, they can supply critical information about the care they receive because they are the direct recipients of that care (Chu & Chu, 1991). Yet unfortunately, some institutions still in the transition from traditional Quality Assurance to CQI aren't making the best use of customer feedback. The result is that those individuals who most need the information gleaned from patients and families never receive it. CQI will not succeed in an atmosphere of lofty idealism where caregivers aren't really connected to those they serve.

AN IMPORTANT OUTCOME INDICATOR

Studies on patient satisfaction first appeared in the literature in the middle of this century. With the introduction of CQI into the healthcare system, patient satisfaction surveys were quickly snared as a relatively easy way to gain customer input. However, healthcare managers' perceptions of the value of that data have ranged from very helpful to practically useless, with many questioning the reliability and validity of data generated (Lansky, 1995). An important initial first step is to decide how you plan to use the data, lest you become a victim of DRIP (Data Rich, Information Poor). We are virtually drowning in data. As CQI gains more sophistication, the real challenge will be transforming patient satisfaction data into meaningful change at various stages of the process improvement cycle (Lansky, 1995).

While patient satisfaction data should never be the single means for evaluating quality of care, they are important monitoring and evaluation methodologies (Eriksen, 1987; Rempusheski, Chamberlain, & Picard, 1988; McDaniel & Nash, 1990). Healthcare organizations are finally returning to the idea that they serve customers. Part of analyzing patient satisfaction data is that caregivers join forces to meet common organizational objectives and to identify opportunities for improving care, rather than "coming to work each day with a little brick or mortar, and trying to build the wall around themselves and their departments a little higher" (Arnold, 1993, p. 81).

Never discount your customers' input. So often we healthcare providers see only what we're looking for, even in our quality improvement programs. Customer survey findings are a "report card" of sorts, pointing us to our problems, and helping us to understand healthcare through their eyes and ultimately to improve outcomes.

THE DOLLAR VALUE OF PATIENT SATISFACTION

Patient dissatisfaction dramatically decreases an organization's economic bottom line (Press, Ganey, & Malone, 1991). Intense competition has jolted many healthcare organizations into taking customer satisfaction more seriously, although many experts still believe it has not yet been accorded the attention it deserves. Plain and simple, we remember businesses that treat us well and those that treat us poorly. Once considered soft data, patient satisfaction findings are now right up there with hard financial measurement data when it comes to making important organizational decisions (Greene, 1994). It is one of the most cost-effective and least invasive ways to keep your finger on the ever-fluctuating pulse of your facility, and will help you make better decisions regarding allocation of limited resources (Press, Ganey Associates, Inc., 1992).

Average is as close to the bottom as it is to the top. "We don't want patients to be just satisfied," says Linde Howell, Manager of Assessment Services for SunHealth Alliance in Charlotte, North Carolina. "We want them to be delighted with services and loyal to the organization" (Greene, 1994).

Customers—satisfied or not—tell their stories to anyone who will listen, and this ultimately affects an organization's competitiveness, even continuation of third-party contracts. Patients say the darndest things, but better they say them to us, and the sooner the better. A sign posted at H&R Block sums up the philosophy of the business world: "Satisfied with our service? Tell a friend. If you're not, tell us."

THE VOICE OF THE CUSTOMER

Customer satisfaction surveys allow patients to have a greater voice in both the design and delivery of healthcare services, and are an important form of market research for healthcare organizations.

Yet in a 1992 article, "The Customer's Voice in Healthcare," Schroeder noted that only 26% of hospitals view customer input as vitally important in strategic planning. Far too often, healthcare is based on providers' needs and not the consumers' (Turner & Matthews, 1991). "We're the experts and we know what they need" is an outdated philosophy.

But we will never fully know our customers by the comments entered on a patient satisfaction survey. Watch for letters to the newspaper editor about your facility. Really pay attention to your customers. At the close of the day or shift, take a little time with your coworkers to evaluate how well you've met customer needs. Are you improving? Seek first to understand, then to be understood.

It's advisable to try to assess an individual's past experiences with the healthcare system. If a patient comes to the E.R. with chest pain and, 6 months before, their father died in your E.R., they're far more likely to overreact in that setting. Furthermore, it's impossible to fully understand the stress generated by family, friends, job, and finances, as well as plain old fear and anxiety that may complicate perceptions of care provided. If this is the case, take a level-headed approach and adjust your own expectations, balancing idealism with realism.

"The customer may not always be right, but the customer is always the customer," says a customer service representative. "They are the only ones who can assess their personal experience with healthcare. Focus on the issue at hand, and not who is 'right'." It sometimes helps to imagine the problem already solved, then look back to the steps it would have likely taken to resolve it, recommend Baber and Waymon (1994). And focus primarily on solutions, not the people responsible for the problem.

PATIENT FOCUS GROUPS

Focus groups are an increasingly popular method of obtaining customer feedback, and have introduced a new kind of data into the CQI process. Consider establishing a focus group to gain an even better understanding of what it's like to be a patient at your facility (Quinn, 1992) and what's important to customers. Such an endeavor provides an excellent opportunity to identify trends in what patients really want from your facility and to improve your organization's overall performance.

Focus groups are typically comprised of 8-12 patients and/or family members (Editor, 1995) to solicit their viewpoint for future organizational decision making and program evaluation, and to increase management's sensitivity to customer concerns. A focus group can be designed to look at particular issues such as: what nurses can do to make you feel they are concerned and caring (Smith, Scammon, & Beck, 1995), environmental and aesthetic preferences, or patient-perceived effectiveness of a particular intervention or change in healthcare delivery. At one small 50-bed hospital in Colorado, a patient care team (which included staff from all clinical services and quality improvement personnel) organized focus groups to improve communication between direct care providers, support staff, and the patient representative (Dugar, 1995).

In an article on patient-driven systems, Adele Pike, a clinical nurse specialist in surgical nursing, tells about a focus group her hospital hosted over informal suppers. "How profound an experience it was," she said, "to see patients we cared for sitting around the table, wearing their street clothes, talking to us as the people they really are, rather than as patients transformed by disease. For all our talk about understanding patients and collaborating with them, this was the experience that really stretched us the most" (Gordon, 1994, p. 8).

The focus group's moderator should be skilled in group process to stay on target and appropriately manage any emotionally charged issues. Sessions should follow a structured format, and it may be helpful to send a letter to participants in advance detailing the purpose of the meeting, and to clarify arrangements for transportation and token compensation.

Consumers generally find focus groups to be a positive experience which can benefit future patients. And, unlike healthcare workers too often bound by bureaucracy, they can dream of the way things *could* be. Staff, in exchange, gain valuable qualitative data and are reminded that patients and families are partners—not passive recipients—of care (Ziegenfuss & O'Rourke, 1995). Focus groups can also help to design or pretest your patient satisfaction questionnaire, pointing out any areas of confusion (Madson, 1994).

PATIENT SATISFACTION QUESTIONNAIRE CONSTRUCTION AND USE

Not all patient satisfaction questionnaires are created equal. "You are only as good as your tool," emphasizes a Quality Improvement Coordinator for a large inner-city hospital. The goal of a patient satisfaction instrument is to capture the heart of a patient's experience with the healthcare system, and provide information that will help providers plan and implement outcome-based care. Ideally, questions should dovetail with an organization's mission, vision, and values, as well as short- and long-term goals.

Press, Ganey Associates, Inc. (1992) have identified the following dos and don'ts for designing and implementing a patient satisfaction survey, which are worthy of consideration:

- Make sure your instrument is designed and tested by staff with some training in survey research methodology.

- Derive questions from patients, particularly patient focus groups. Questions must reflect issues of importance to patients, rather than administrators.

- Keep the instrument to both sides of one sheet of paper, regular or legal size. [Many organizations use legal-size paper folded in half to make a four-page booklet.]

- Don't use glossy paper or pastel inks.

- Use a five-point scale for the entire instrument. Never mix scales (i.e., "good–bad," "satisfied–dissatisfied," "yes-no," etc.). The results can't be compared.

- Use wording the patients use: "E.R." not "E.D.," etc.

- Never put propaganda on the instrument. No photos of dedicated nurses.

- Use a separate, short, straightforward cover letter with no hype about your great hospital, its lofty goals and staff. Return address should be to "Director, Patient Relations" or other non-intimidating title.

- Never distribute instruments to patients while they are still in the hospital.

- Mail questionnaires to patients within a day or two of discharge. Mail-out yields up to 30% or more return rate. Handout at discharge yields 5%–15% return.

- Phone surveys are much more expensive to maintain on a continuing basis. They are best used to delve deeper into problems that mail-out instruments or patient complaints have revealed.

- Provide space for written comments after each questionnaire section, rather than once, at the end of the instrument.

- For analysis, convert your five-point scale to a 0-100 scale, and work with mean scores for each item, rather than simplistic breakdown of percentage of responses (e.g., 53% very satisfied, 17% satisfied, etc.).

- Use factor analysis and correlation coefficients to derive statistics that indicate the relative importance of each question and section to overall patient satisfaction.*

Some organizations establish a task force to review tools in the literature and to design a facility-specific questionnaire. The unique cultural, educational, and language characteristics of the patient population under study should always be taken into con-

*Copyright 1992 Press, Ganey Associates, Inc. Used with permission.

sideration. Some questions to consider are: Will patients likely be able to understand the questions? What is the specific goal of your survey? Ferguson and Ferguson (1983) stress that the purpose of such surveys is to elicit information that the patient is better qualified than anyone else to tell us. Patients must view the exercise as purposeful, for, like us, they are easily put off by work they perceive as meaningless.

The manner in which questions are worded (open-ended versus a rating scale of very poor to very good versus yes/no) will significantly affect the type and quality of responses. Yes/no and scaled formats provide data for statistical evaluation and graphic presentation, and minimize the time it requires to complete the survey. Open-ended questions get at the heart of patients' deeper concerns, put a real person behind the numbers, and give you a clue to the stories your patients are telling your current and potential future customers.

Imagine you're standing in line at the supermarket and an old friend tells you that the care at Dr. France's office was "fair." Wouldn't you want to know more, especially if your daughter has an appointment to see Dr. France for the first time the following week? But if your friend tells you she had to wait three hours, the office staff was rude and inconsiderate, and Dr. France herself skirted her questions, you have real flesh and blood examples of the personality of the place. You may choose to believe the staff at Dr. France's office were just having a bad day, but you will have more data on which to make that assumption.

And so it is with customer satisfaction data. If we obtain vague data, at best we vaguely address the problem, and arrive at a vague solution. A combined approach (where comments are solicited) will give you both quantitative and qualitative data.

How Was the Questionnaire Completed?

If a patient completes a satisfaction survey soon after undergoing surgery or a procedure where sedatives were administered, this should be taken into account when evaluating responses. Stress and anxiety may also affect perceptions and recall (Leino-Kilpi &

Vuorenheimo, 1993). Was the respondent under the influence of alcohol or other mind-altering substances? This could also pollute the data.

Did the patient complete the form over a period of several days? If so, and their medical condition and level of pain or hope changed significantly, this will influence findings. Be mindful that a dependent patient who is encouraged to participate in self-care activities may report dissatisfaction with healthcare, even though (and perhaps, because) extensive education and discharge planning efforts were instituted (Eriksen, 1987).

There is no guarantee that a questionnaire was even completed by the recipient of care. When you receive a survey in your mailbox about your favorite brand of cereal, if you don't view it as all that important, might you not let your 12-year-old son fill in the blanks? How do we know that a patient's 10-year-old grandson didn't complete her satisfaction survey just for the fun of it? And those blistering comments on Mr. Galloway's survey that don't sound a thing like him—maybe they aren't his at all. It's possible that his daughter, who just had a conflict with her own doctor, read you the riot act to rid her own frustrations. That's why we further investigate any pertinent concerns and look for trends.

All patient should have the opportunity to evaluate the care without fear that such information will be used against them. But data is only as meaningful as the tool is reliable and valid (McDaniel & Nash, 1990).

ASSESS SATISFACTION ON MANY LEVELS

Patient satisfaction can be assessed by mail, face-to-face or telephone interviews, or a combination of all these methods (Kelly-Heidenthal, 1992). Each has its inherent strengths and weaknesses, and response rates are influenced by the approach used.

Telephone interviews allow you to obtain a considerable amount of information in a relatively short period of time, provided you are able to track down that individual. But if you caught them in the middle of something or they are annoyed with their next-door neighbor for running the lawn mower while they are trying to sleep, this will skew results.

One situation where the telephone interview is a superior assessment tool is for the patient who has undergone an outpatient surgery or diagnostic test. An individual involved in this care who has already established rapport with the patient and family can telephone them to ask if they are experiencing any complications, if they need any clarification of information presented (Johnson & Wilson, 1984), if they were satisfied with their care, and how future service could be improved.

"If there was a misunderstanding, this is a wonderful time to smooth any ruffled feathers," says Sandra, a nurse who assists with outpatient G.I. procedures. "You can find out so much by what appears to them to just be chitchat. We'll be talking about their little pooch, and the next thing I know they're telling me they got light-headed when they walked to the bathroom. That, of course, leads to the question, 'Have you had any blood in your stool?'—a question that might be a bit awkward if asked out of the blue over the phone. And patients always remember that you called them at home to check on them. I think it's a carryover from the old country doctor days."

Interviews conducted on-site (sometimes in the form of an exit interview) have the best response rate because you have a captive audience. But patients may be reluctant to discuss their true concerns for fear of reprisal, and such an approach is quite labor intensive.

Face-to-face and phone interviews are extremely dependent on both the skill of the interviewer and the patient's feelings about the interviewer. If Cathy, the dear nurse who took such wonderful care of you after your hysterectomy, is asking you questions, you may be less likely to tell her your hospital experience as a whole didn't meet your expectations. You won't want to take a chance on her taking it personally and hurting her feelings.

Don't fall into the trap of assuming that "just about anyone" can solicit or evaluate patient satisfaction data. It should be an individual who has expertise in the interviewing process and who has an understanding of clinical and administrative issues, as well as how to initiate referrals. Inevitably questions will arise, and if the person continuously answers, "I'm sorry, I don't know," confidence will be broken and the respondent may not answer the remaining questions as seriously or thoroughly. You don't want your customers to perceive that this is a necessary evil, something we have to get over with. As in all areas, they usually take their cues from us.

We are no longer a world who is fond of communicating via the written word. People don't write notes and letters even to loved ones like they used to. When someone takes the time to write long narratives about their care, take them seriously.

DEMOGRAPHIC DATA

Don't collect demographic information you don't need just because you think you should be asking it. If in your strategic planning you are considering offering support groups for patients with your facility's top chronic illness DRGs, it may be appropriate to ask questions related to social interests and transportation. Be careful, though, that such questions don't appear to be intrusive. Rather let your customer know that you are in the process of designing additional services to address their special needs.

When assessing sensitive demographic data, such as those related to finances, word questions carefully and try not to place them at the beginning of a survey. As one elderly man said, "They asked me how much money my wife and I had saved. I peeled the uncancelled stamp off their envelope and threw their survey in the trash. We fork out $600.00 a month for prescriptions and I'm not taking a chance on them confiscating our social security checks. We saved for a rainy day and now we're in the middle of a thunder storm. You just can't trust people like you used to."

UNANSWERED QUESTIONS AND UNQUESTIONED ANSWERS

If you fail to ask the right questions in the right manner, you won't tap into the real issues that concern your customers (Lytle, 1993). A good analogy for this is the patient with a beginning pressure ulcer. On the surface, the patient's skin may merely appear inflamed and the skin integrity may only be slightly compromised. As a nurse, you can bask in the security that this is a minimal problem, or recognize that such a situation likely represents only the tip of the iceberg. Underneath the surface, there is damage not evident to the casual observer. Likewise, what about satisfaction surveys that aren't returned at all?

SHARE RESULTS WITH STAFF

To truly understand the lessons inherent in patient satisfaction data, survey results should be analyzed in light of the organization's overall objectives (Butcher, 1994). Communicate findings to appropriate caregivers so that changes in the day-to-day functioning of the institution/department are based on what your customers tell you (Strasen, 1988). Even staff who don't have direct patient contact should be included, as this is a superb way to help them care about customers they may never actually see.

Baggett (1994) emphasizes that if departments aren't communicating with each other effectively, you can be certain they aren't communicating well with their customers either. Patients and families can tell when we work well together as a team (Treat Everyone As Me), and when the environment is a supportive, cohesive one. In examining patient satisfaction findings, we should always be asking ourselves and each other: "Are we communicating so that everyone comes together for the care of our patients?"

Patient satisfaction in some institutions is the focus of interdisciplinary CQI teams to enhance organizational performance. An excellent example of this is at Hospital Corporation of America (HCA) hospitals, where an ingenious system is in place that makes use of computer technology to assess on-site customer reactions to their healthcare experience. Patients enter their responses in a personal computer. Data analysis by time of day, department, and day of the week can give the organization an up-to-date view of whether inpatients or outpatients perceive their needs are being met. Quality improvement teams then analyze data and present findings to staff, and identify opportunities to improve care (Koska, 1992).

Improving organizational performance is based on having good data and using it to the best advantage. What are you doing with your patient satisfaction data? Do the right people have the customer input they need to make informed decisions? Are organizational decisions based on what your customers are telling you? These are questions the JCAHO is asking as well when they survey hospitals. Employees, patients, and families are now even interviewed by surveyors to determine perceptions of care.

PERILS AND PITFALLS

While the importance of measuring patient satisfaction is gaining ground across the country in healthcare, many methodologies are outdated. Irwin Press, Ph.D., a co-director of Press, Ganey Associates, Inc., one of the nation's largest patient satisfaction monitoring firms, makes this observation:

> Unfortunately, many hospitals still utilize surveys that produce data which are meaningless for management. In many cases, questions and response scales are skewed towards positive responses, not towards identifying problem areas. Even those hospitals with well-designed questionnaires may lack the ability to produce statistical analyses and reports for individual departments or nursing units or to prepare reports in a timely manner. (Press, Ganey Associates, Inc., 1994)

Many tools only assess superficial issues—"How was the food?" "How did the nurses treat you?" Too many organizations measure what's easy to measure, not what they should be measuring ... what will ultimately help the customer (Whiteley, 1991).

Because of the tremendous variability in patient satisfaction assessment tools, it's next to impossible to compare how one agency stands up against another (Greene, 1994). You may find the services of an outside consultation firm invaluable in designing a questionnaire and in analyzing the findings. Press's agency, for example, provides satisfaction surveys for a myriad of inpatient and outpatient settings, and processes more than 250,000 surveys quarterly. A representative sample and a reasonable response rate are critical to having meaningful data. Ideally you should be able to compare your findings with national benchmarks of comparable facilities and patient populations.

READING THE CUSTOMER'S MIND

Have you ever, during the holidays, hinted to your mother or husband about a new sweater you spotted at a department store? You'd really like to find it gift-wrapped under the tree on Christmas morning. But to come right out and ask for it, well that's just a little too pushy. Besides, it's far more impressive when someone picks up on your hints and grants you your heart's desire.

Without consciously trying to play games, our patients do a similar thing. They drop hints about how care and services could be better, but they rarely come right out and ask for them. Many patients don't verbalize their concerns unsolicited to staff.

That's why it's helpful for your hospital's patient representative to visit every patient as soon after admission as possible, to communicate the institution's procedure for expressing problems and concerns. And visits during hospitalization can bring issues to light early on while they are still fresh in the patient's mind (Press, 1984). For we caregivers are just like mothers and husbands; in our busy lives and with all our distractions, we often pass by even not-so-subtle hints.

LOOK AT EMPLOYEE MORALE

There's no question that patient satisfaction data will point you to problems of employee morale within your organization (Greene, 1994). Patients pick up on dissension, and in turn employees project their own dissatisfaction onto customers. Does your agency reward employees who excel in making customers happy? Many industries do. Or do employees get the sense that no one notices when you go the extra mile for a customer, or worse yet discourage it?

"We counsel nurses for medication errors," says Barbara, a pediatrics nurse, "and that's appropriate. But what about disciplining nurses for treating patients and families badly?" Staff should be empowered to serve customers, and data on customer satisfaction should be communicated to them.

FOLLOW-UP WITH CUSTOMERS ON DOWN THE ROAD

If you really want to know what customers remember, place a call a year later to assess what nursing interventions were most helpful or frustrating. If you work on an oncology or hospice unit, you might want to incorporate this into your bereavement support program. A telephone call on the anniversary of a loved one's death can be quite meaningful, especially when it comes from someone who cared for them during their final days. And family members are usually more than pleased to offer insight which will improve the care of other patients.

SATISFACTION GUARANTEED

There's a great story about Bill Arnold, President of Centennial Medical Center in Nashville, Tennessee. In showcasing his innovative approach to participatory leadership, author Nancy Austin (1991, p. 42) wrote: "One of his first acts at Centennial was to shatter sacrosanct management tradition by yanking his office door from its hinges and suspending it from the lobby ceiling to underscore his commitment to an open-door policy."

In healthcare, we need open doors at every turn. We've traveled too far away from each other. Healthcare administrators, providers, and customers need to really listen to each other and to their customers. And when a concern is expressed, we need to check it out, because a concern voiced by one individual is likely perceived similarly by others. As experience has proven, technology only takes us so far. It's the human dimension in satisfying customers that really tips the balance.

Listen, and ask why, why, why? And keep listening, because customers' needs change every day. This is the era of the customer, and they will tell us what they want and need if we'll only pay attention. The goal for customer service is 100% customer satisfaction (Baggett, 1994). Yet even if our customers are satisfied, we should never be. There are always opportunities to improve care and services.

References

Arnold, W. III. (1993). The leader's role in implementing quality improvement: Walking the talk. *QRB, 19*(3), 79-82.

Austin, N. K. (1991, Nov.). Wacky management ideas that work. *Working Woman,* 42-45.

Baber, A., & Waymon, L. (1994, Aug./Sep./Oct.). Win-win negotiation. *Carlson Voyager,* 30-31.

Baggett, B. (1994). *Satisfaction guaranteed.* Nashville: Rutledge Hill Press.

Butcher, A. H. (1994). Supervisors matter more than you think: Components of a mission-centered organizational climate. *Hospitals and Health Services Administration, 39*(4), 505-520.

Chu, L. K., & Chu, G. S. F. (1991). Feedback and efficiency: A staff development model. *Nursing Management, 22*(2), 28-31.

Dugar, B. (1995). Implementing CQI on a budget: A small hospital's story. *Journal of Quality Improvement, 21*(2), 57-69.

Editor. (1995). Patient's perspective: Using patient input in a cycle for performance improvement. *Journal of Quality Improvement, 21*(2), 87-96.

Eriksen, L. R. (1987). Patient satisfaction: An indicator of nursing care quality? *Nursing Management, 18*(7), 31-35.

Ferguson, G., & Ferguson, W. F. (1983). As patients see us. *Nursing Management, 14*(8), 20-21.

Gelmon, S. B., & Baker, G. R. (1995). Incorporating quality improvement in health administration curriculum. *The Journal of Health Administration Education, 13*(1), 91-106.

Gordon, S. (1994, June). Inside the patient-driven system. *Critical Care Nurse* (supplement), 2-28.

Greene, J. (1994, July 18). Competition for patients spurs hospitals' concern for serving the customer. *Modern Health Care,* 30-34.

JCAHO. (1994). *The Joint Commission 1995 comprehensive accreditation manual for hospitals. Volume I: Standards.* Oakbrook Terrace, IL: Author.

Johnson, S., & Wilson, L. (1984). *The one minute sales person.* New York: Avon Books.

Kelly-Heidenthal, P. (1992). Are your patients satisfied? *Nursing Quality Connection, 1*(5).

Koska, M. T. (1992, Nov. 5). Surveying customer needs, not satisfaction, is crucial to CQI. *Hospitals,* 50-53.

Lansky, D. (1995). Quality improvement in health care: The year behind, the year ahead. *Journal of Quality Improvement, 21*(1), 32-43.

Leino-Kilpi, H., & Vuorenheimo, J. (1993). Perioperative nursing care quality. *AORN Journal, 57*(5), 1061-1071.

Lytle, J. F. (1993). *What do your customers really want?* Chicago, IL: Probus Publishing Co.

Madson, S. K. (1994). Tips for designing a client satisfaction tool. *Nursing Quality Connection, 3*(6), 7.

McDaniel, C., & Nash, J. G. (1990). Compendium of instruments measuring patient satisfaction with nursing care. *Quality Review Bulletin, 16*(5), 182-188.

Press, Ganey Associates, Inc. (1994). *Patient satisfaction measurement: A vital management tool.* South Bend, IN: Author.

Press, Ganey Associates, Inc. (1992). *The satisfaction report.* South Bend, IN: Author.

Press, I., Ganey, R.F., & Malone, M.P. (1991, Feb.). Satisfied patients can spell financial well-being. *Healthcare Financial Management,* 34-42.

Press, I. (1984, April). The predisposition to file claims: The patient's perspective. *Law, Medicine and Health Care,* 53-62.

Quinn, D. (1992). Principles of data collection applied to customer knowledge. *JHQ, 14*(6), 24-36.

Rempusheski, V. F., Chamberlain, S. L., & Picard, H. B. (1988). Expected and received care: Patient perceptions. *Nursing Administration Quarterly, 12*(3), 42-50.

Schroeder, P. (1992). The customer's voice in health care. *Nursing Quality Connection, 2*(3), 3.

Shortell, S. M. (1995). Assessing the evidence on CQI: Is the glass half empty or half full? *Hospital and Health Services Administration, 40*(1), 4-24.

Smith, J. A., Scammon, D. L., & Beck, S. L. (1995). Using patient focus groups for new patient services. *Journal of Quality Improvement, 21*(1), 22-31.

Strasen, L. (1988). Incorporating patient satisfaction standards into quality of care measures. *Journal of Nursing Administration, 18*(11), 5-6.

Turner, J. T., & Matthews, K. A. (1991, Summer). Measuring adolescent satisfaction with nursing care in an ambulatory setting. *The ABNF Journal,* 48-52.

Whiteley, R. C. (1991). *The customer driven company: Moving from talk to action.* Reading, MA: Addison-Wesley Publishing Co.

Ziegenfuss, J. T., & O'Rourke, P. (1995). Ombudsmen, patient complaints, and total quality management: An examination of fit. *Journal of Quality Improvement, 21*(3), 133-142.

Chapter 9

BE KIND TO YOURSELF AND YOUR COWORKERS

A Plan for Enhanced Morale and Patient Satisfaction

Unless someone like you cares a whole awful lot,
nothing is going to get better. It's not.
— Dr. Seuss (Geisel & Geisel, 1971)

L inda, a staff nurse on a busy surgical unit, crawls out of bed at 5 AM every morning, 2 hours before her husband Tom and two children see the light of day. There's breakfast to prepare ("to give my family a good start"), a couple of loads of laundry to toss in the washer, and the apartment to tidy up. Once she's showered, pulled on her uniform, and completed her early morning chores, she feeds her family, dresses her kids, and drops them off at day care on her way to the hospital.

With the kisses of two toddlers still wet on her cheek, Linda can't help but count her blessings. A family she loves and a profession she's dreamed of since she was her own tiny Amy's age: nursing. She'd be caring for the patients on team two today. How she'd grown attached to Mr. Smithers, who'd undergone a colostomy this admission. Today, he'd be discharged home, more accepting of his illness and able to care for his stoma, at least in part, thanks to her.

Linda swelled with pride over her family and her job. *I juggle it all pretty well,* she thought as she headed toward the nurses' station. *Of course, that doesn't leave much time for me, but my time will come later when the kids are grown. I'm thankful to even have a job with all this talk of layoffs, mergers, and down-sizing.* Just then, Janice, the night nurse, lashed out at her in front of a group of new nursing students. "We're sick and tired of dealing with your messes, Linda. For the second night in a row, evenings has found a dirty bed on your team. When are you going to get your act together?"

When are you going to get your act together? The words echoed in Linda's mind the whole day, chipping away at her confidence. Only an hour before, she'd felt equipped to take on the day with enthusiasm. But a coworker's hasty remark changed all that.

Or did it?

In an average lifetime, the average American spends 70,696 hours working (Heymann, 1991). No one has ventured to estimate how many medications administered, I.V.s started, or patients educated—that adds up to for the average nurse. But the fact remains, we spend one third of our working lives at our place of employment. Why then are we so often unkind to each other? And, even more pressing, why don't we treat ourselves with the same love and consideration we accord our families and patients?

There's no question that patients and visitors can immediately sense a medical environment where the staff at best tolerate each other. Such an atmosphere directly affects customer satisfaction and decreases productivity and personnel morale (Brown, Nelson, Bronkesh, & Wood, 1993).

Have you ever visited a home where the children cowered in a corner while the adults argued? The kids' basic need for security was being challenged. The same thing happens when our patients observe us fussing with each other over some small detail, or bad-mouthing a colleague, superior, or staff member from another department behind their back. How secure can you really feel about competence and care in an environment like that? And while *we* may soon forget words uttered in haste, patients—our customers—may well remember them every time they seek care at our facility. How much better to be generous with gentleness.

COWORKERS ARE OUR INTERNAL CUSTOMERS

"People have not been conditioned or encouraged to treat people inside of their own organization as well as they treat customers outside," says Scott (1991, p. 1). "Yet no one works alone. Satisfying internal people provides a vital link in the chain that leads to satisfying customers outside of the organization." This attitude should be introduced to nursing students from day one, and caring behaviors modeled in the instructor–student relationship.

It's increasingly recognized that nurses who first address their own personal needs are clearly more effective in helping patients. "We are taught to sacrifice and suffer for the good of those around us, yet when it comes to our own self-care, I wonder how many of us sacrifice that as well?" asks Caryn Summers (1994, p. 94).

Furthermore, coworkers who sincerely care for and about each other promote an atmosphere of warmth, collaboration, professional accountability, and balance that patients perceive as a safe environment of caring. It's a fact that some nursing departments resemble a dysfunctional family. There's the rescuer (we typically have several of them), the victim (enough of those, too), the peacemaker (we usually really like them), and don't forget the unit mascot.

There's much to learn about what makes a family strong. A *Family Circle* Family Index (1993) came up with seven key characteristics, more than half of which have implications for nursing:

- They make time for relaxation.

- They know how to express anger without hurt feelings.

- They (adults) do their quarreling privately.

- They feel connected to their community.

CARING FOR EACH OTHER

How often have you heard nurses say: "We're our own worst enemy" . . . "Nursing is the only profession that eats its young" . . . "Doctors stick together, even when one of them is wrong, but not us" . . . "They drive everyone off that's good around here" . . . "I've never seen anything like it, the way nurses go after each other. For nurturers, they sure are cutthroats."

We've become a very warped profession. Sadly, as Walt Kelly, the creator of the philosophical Pogo comic strip, once observed, "We have met the enemy and he is us."

A patient with degenerative joint disease observes: "There's nothing as poignant as a truly caring nurse and nothing as exasperating as one who appears not to care." What potential nurses have for creating a truly therapeutic environment . . . to face each new day, as one cancer patient suggests, putting into each letter, each phone call, each dish washed, a full measure of love (McFarland, 1993). But what we do flows from who we are inside, and if we don't care for ourselves and each other, we have little to give.

BREAKING THE DESTRUCTIVE CYCLE

When people have been hurt, observes Larry Crabb (1990), they invest most of their energy seeing to it that they don't get hurt again. The investment of energy in counterproductive or self-sabotaging behavior is a symptom of one of nursing's biggest problems, and adversely affects customer satisfaction. Taking care of ourselves is a primary preventive measure against burnout that inevitably occurs when we put others' needs first and neglect our own, says Summers (1994).

Nothing breaks that vicious cycle like the gift of encouragement. Nursing, the single largest group of healthcare providers, is a wounded profession. A transformation, however, won't take place on a national level, at the state level, or even at an organizational level. It must begin in the heart of every nurse who determines to make the future of nursing as caring a place for its own sake as for those we serve.

When Presbyterian-St. Luke's Medical Center in Chicago implemented Total Quality Management, it found the single most significant byproduct to be the improved attitude of employees toward their coworkers. "The recognition of fellow employees as 'customers' has created a new awareness and willingness to meet their expectations," they said. "The result is more satisfied and effective employees and, ultimately, more satisfied external customers" (Melum & Sinioris, 1989, p. 80). Clearly, empowerment of staff and the shared accountability inherent in a team approach to healthcare is critical to an organizational culture of continuous quality improvement (Brodeur, 1995).

With the disconcerting changes in healthcare at every turn, nursing is at a crossroads. We can vow to infuse our clinical settings with a transfusion of kindness—for ourselves, those we care for, and our coworkers. To do so would virtually revolutionize the delivery of healthcare.

NURSING'S GREATEST MOMENTS

Consider what Stephen Nachmanovitch had to say in *Free Play* (1990), a book about the power of improvisation in life and the arts:

> Indeed, many great performances have been recorded, and we are glad to have them. But I think the greatest performances always elude the camera, the tape recorder, the pen. They happen in the middle of the night when the musician plays for one special friend under the moonlight, they happen in the dress rehearsal just before the play opens. (p. 24)

They happen, too, behind a closed door when a night shift nurse holds a frightened patient's hand in a never-to-be-duplicated moment. They happen when a school nurse goes to great lengths to make a referral for a child with a learning disability, even (and most especially) though no one may ever know. They happen when a hospice nurse drives a dying husband to watch his wife of five short years direct the community Christmas pageant. And they happen when an office nurse lets go of a grudge, a nursing instructor gives that struggling student nurse a second chance (and a new beginning), and an Emergency Room nurse looks beyond the seemingly bad attitude of a coworker to see a frustrated single dad.

"If a tree falls in the forest with no one there to hear it, does it make a sound?" (Cook, 1992, p. 22) No one has to witness the memorable moments of nursing for them to change us as individuals and as a profession. Sure, the Joint Commission pays hospitals a visit at least every three years to tell us how we measure up. Your facility may be inspected by still other external reviewing/consulting agencies. And patient satisfaction surveys give us meaningful measurements of how our patients perceive their care. But this is only part of the total quality picture.

LET RESPECT BE YOUR GUIDE

"Treat everyone in the organization with respect and dignity, whether it be the janitor or the president," advises Richard Moran (1993, No. 344). When people feel more trusted and valued, they do better work and can be more spontaneous. A hospice nurse who has a personal history of childhood sexual abuse said: "If the staff know you're trying to take care of them, they'll work harder. If they sense they're being abused, they'll work far less."

Being yourself (within appropriate boundaries, of course) is one way of demonstrating self-respect. Perhaps you've heard nurses say, "When those 'nine-to-fivers' treat us with respect, we can start treating our patients that way." While there shouldn't be an adversarial relationship between staff and administration, respect begins with the individual worker.

Hal Rosenbluth, the CEO of Rosenbluth Travel, a company that experienced a 7500% growth in revenue over a 15-year period, stresses that employees are an organization's internal customers. Focus on your employees because of your customers, he says. His advice is admittedly somewhat controversial: "Companies must put their people—not their customers—first" (Rosenbluth & Peters, 1992, p. 10). Yet as a result, his employees excel at customer service, and the once family business is now a global enterprise.

In these changing healthcare times when nurses—even those with years of valuable experience—have less job security, it's especially unsettling to hear comments like, "If you don't like it, there's 15 people waiting to take your place." A practice such as referring to some employees as "non-essential" during a snow storm can communicate subtle negative messages.

Want a tip? To build respect in your department, first recognize that no one functions in a vacuum. One hospital pharmacist astutely observed: "Nurses work better by themselves than in groups." Team building can be intense, but it's well worth the effort. An activity as simple as all staff members in a physician's office eating lunch together once a month can work wonders in building interdisciplinary respect and camaraderie. Or, consider taking on a special community project such as filling stockings for needy children at Christmas to begin moving in the same direction.

PRAISE IN PUBLIC, CORRECT IN PRIVATE

Have you ever complimented a coworker and seen the mood on your unit magically lighten? We nurses should praise each other, not punish each other. Sadly, too many nurses, used to being belittled at every turn, are uncomfortable with recognition. "Why can't we bring out the best in each other instead of sending 'nasty-grams?'" asks Jane, a nurse on a hectic metabolic unit.

One day I carried what I thought to be a beautiful carved oak rocker out of an antiques store. As I was loading it into my trunk, a competing dealer from across the street yelled, "I see that kindling you just bought." It reminded me of some of the offhand remarks we nurses sometimes make to each other.

"Never correct a co-worker in front of a customer or client ... or anyone else," reminds Moran (1993, No. 152). We've all heard that an unreasonably critical person is most often reflecting their own inadequacies. But that doesn't help when we're the target of humiliating comments. As one staff nurse explains: "When you talk down to another nurse in front of a patient or family, you undermine their future trust in that person. What if that nurse later responds to them in a crisis? You've not only broken their trust, you've also hurt the patient."

Unfortunately, criticism sometimes has its roots in the green-eyed monster, jealousy. It's always easier to critique than create, but it destroys the very heart and soul of nursing. Alice Miller's maxim is food for thought for nurses: "If it is very painful of you to criticize your friends, you are safe in doing it. But if you take the slightest pleasure in it, that is the time to hold your tongue."

KEEP YOUR PERSONAL LIFE IN BALANCE

Many people work diligently on the job, yet smother their nagging discontent with all manner of destructive behaviors like workaholism, excessive drinking, and compulsive behaviors (Pearson, 1991). When you're pulled at every turn, it's difficult to achieve that necessary delicate balance.

But consider this sentiment, the author of which is unknown: "First I was dying to finish high school and start college. And then I was dying to finish college and start working. And then I was dying to marry and have children. And then I was dying for my children to grow old enough for school so I could return to work. And then I was dying to retire. And now, I am dying ... and suddenly I realize I forgot to live."

SAY "YES" TO YOUR DREAMS

Would you believe that in the first 18 years of life, we are told "No," or what we can't do, over 148,000 times (Pearson, 1991)? Give yourself a "Yes I can" message. If it seems foreign to you, be patient. "The mind is slow in unlearning what it has been long in learning" (Seneca).

Nurses hear too many negative, devaluing messages as it is. So much of life is a result of the messages we tell ourselves in private moments. Be kind to yourself and true to your dreams. You deserve the best that life and nursing have to offer.

It's Okay to Be Angry

If you cut yourself off from your feelings, be they love, denial, anger, and so on, you're at greater risk for a myriad of maladies. Anger is like physical pain; it's a symbol something is wrong or out of balance. Just as a bell sounds both alarm and joy, anger—if we're honest with ourselves—can open us up to a whole new dimension of living.

When you hear a nurse remark, "All I have to show for 20 years of nursing is a bad back and varicose veins," that's a sign that individual is experiencing anger. We may call it burnout, depression, resentment, irritation, or whatever, but that doesn't deny the existence of anger nor its impact on our lives.

We have a right to be angry. No one likes to feel used and unappreciated, and many of us do in both our personal and professional lives. "If you act like a doormat, I've discovered people will walk on you," says Jane, a psychiatric clinical nurse specialist. So often nurses are responsive to everyone else's needs, yet deny their own. We're taught to say "sure" to every request. Inside we're numb, and still saying "sure." We feel like we're never doing enough and never doing it well enough. And all too often doing comes at the expense of feeling.

Give yourself permission to feel. Feeling anger is neither right nor wrong. It simply is. If we don't assert ourselves, we pay a dear price in terms of ill health and damage to our spirit. Our credo is "first do no harm." That goes for nurses, too.

Sometimes, however, we have difficulty in making our needs known. Ann, a hospice supervisor, once noticed that her usually calm and supportive staff were "acting out." "Before I confronted the issue, I reviewed our patient mortality statistics for the past month and realized we'd had 40 deaths. My nurses were grieving, and I called a series of staff meetings to help them come to grips with their feelings of 'Why? Why? Why?'"

Sally, a nurse office manager for a group of E.N.T. specialists, says: "I'm learning to ask directly for what I need, rather than hoping others will second-guess me. If I've had a bad day, I'll call my husband and say, 'I need to go out for dinner and unload on you. It's time for a pity party.' Then he knows what I expect, and I don't have to play games. I find I'm much less angry when I take control of my life like that."

The Danger of Detachment

Most of us have gotten especially close to a patient at some time in our careers, and then gone through a period of profound grief when that patient died. "I lost a patient with ovarian cancer who had a daughter the same age as mine," remembers Amy. "It was absolutely terrible. I grieved my heart out. So I decided that would never happen to me again and I began to detach myself from my work. Then a very wise social worker pointed out to me the importance of experiencing a whole range of emotions. She helped me to see when I block out feelings of anger, grief, and loss, I also separate myself from the love all around me. I've learned it's better in the long run to be open and honest—even if it does sometimes make me more vulnerable."

"My daughter was born premature, and they had to put in a feeding tube," remembers Carole. "I noticed my baby's legs were flinching and I asked, 'Does that hurt?' I still get sick at my stomach when I think of what the nurse said: 'I don't know. I've never had one, and I'm not a baby.'"

Sometimes we distance ourselves by referring to patients as "the chest pain in bed three" or the "leukemic in 221." It makes you wonder what kind of message we're communicating to our customers. We desperately need to connect as human beings. Do everything you can to remove distance that divides hurting hearts.

Forget Who Gets the Credit

"One thing I'm learning about nursing is that when you give input, no one really uses it, or at best they discount it," says Jim, a recent graduate. "It gives the message you're worthless." For some reason, it's difficult for many nurses to share expertise and resources. If we'd only realize that no one is ever another individual's competition, maybe we'd not be so tight with our information.

Why can't we rejoice in others' successes rather than quip, "I could've done better than that." Yes, you probably could've, but you didn't at that point in time. It's good to remember that the smallest deed is better than the grandest intention.

Think for a moment. Hasn't there been a background nurse in your career? One who silently spread seeds of kindness without fretting over who got the credit? Like the family who plants a new apple tree even though they're going to move across the country in a year, let's invest in a future we may not actually see. In the end, there's no true satisfaction for any of us unless there's satisfaction for all of us.

GET TO KNOW YOURSELF

Take time to listen to your life and get to know yourself. But examine yourself with a mirror, not a magnifying glass. One secret to finding nursing rewarding is to build in time for solitude, for silencing the endless chatter in our heads. Give yourself a rich inner life. Don't neglect your soul.

Some nurses have found that journaling is a practice that helps them get in touch with themselves. Here's a secret place where you can explore your feelings and learn to better trust your judgment; where you can record and later reflect on small spurts of growth that might go unnoticed. Resist the urge to "pretty up" your entries, however. "What is, is; what ain't, ain't," as one nurse says.

A gentleman with cancer who turned his journal entries into an insightful book of meditations made this observation:

> There's a temptation to go back and rewrite the meditations of the early days and the chemo days and the down days, to give them the benefit of the long view. I've not yielded to that temptation, though. At each of those steps, the way it is is the way it is. When you're there, you're there. That's okay. (McFarland, 1993, p. xviii)

Get to know yourself. And like yourself *now,* not when you lose 20 pounds, save more money, are praised by your peers, or secure a better job. It will add to your personal job satisfaction and to customer satisfaction, because who you are flows out of everything you say and do. Your first customer is yourself: until you're good to yourself, you can't be good to anyone else.

FACE YOUR DISCOMFORT

Change, it is said, is to be bruised in a new place. We don't usually make changes in our lives until we face up to the fact that something is wrong. The monumental changes in healthcare point to a system that is careening out of control.

The stress of being all things to all people in all situations is taking a heavy, tragic toll on the profession of nursing. Additionally, many nurses come from dysfunctional families where alcoholism or physical, emotional, or sexual abuse have forever colored their lives. Those who have encountered the destruction of abusive relationships may fall into the trap of erroneously thinking they are personally responsible for all the future hurts that come their way (Buhler, 1991). Not so. Facing your discomfort and personal pain doesn't mean blaming yourself for it.

When you experience a death or disappointment on your nursing unit, support each other. Take time to ask, "What did that death trigger in my coworker who recently lost her father?"

SURROUND YOURSELF WITH ENCOURAGING PEOPLE

A young terminally ill mother commented on how she felt completely overwhelmed at the thought of leaving her three children and husband behind. "I believed there was nothing I could do to help my despair, and then an idea came to me. I'd form an encouragement team. People who constantly got me down wouldn't be a part of my 'team'."

Of course, nurses can't really eliminate all negative forces from their lives. But they can surround themselves with the voice of encouragement, not people who are threatened by growth and change. "All it takes is one nurse coming to work with a bad attitude to affect the whole department," says Sarah, a unit manager. "It trickles down to patients, too."

How can we really be caregivers if no one cares for us? So often we're unaware of each other's pain, yet wonderful things happen when nurses care for and about each other. "I was diagnosed with diabetes during my first pregnancy," remembers a nurse, "and one of the nursing assistants baked me a tin of diabetic cookies. It was one of the sweetest things anyone has ever done for me; to think he cared enough to take the time. I treated my patients, my coworkers, and my own family with an extra measure of kindness that entire day because of his gift."

TAKE TIME TO PLAY

There's an old adage: When you work, work; when you play, play. "Healthcare workers need to lighten up a little," observes a patient who was hospitalized for an extended period of time. We need to take our work seriously, but ourselves less seriously. Step away from your everyday self and celebrate. Now.

NURTURE YOURSELF

How do you treat someone you dearly love? Treat yourself that way. For wherever you go, you take yourself with you. How about traveling with your best self? When you feel good about yourself, the quality of care you deliver is higher.

Nurses continue to drive themselves when their personal gas tanks are on empty. We're natural nurturers, but we can't continue to give when our inner selves are depleted. As the mountain sage said: "You can't give what you ain't got no more than you can come back from where you ain't been."

How do you replenish yourself on and off the job? Do you carve out a niche of time just for you on your day off? Are you giving yourself enough comforts? Do you take your scheduled breaks at work? Only when we're nurtured from within can we reach out to others and maintain appropriate boundaries. So often we settle for leftovers and don't question that we deserve better. It's like the missionary who received a "CARE" package containing used tea bags and felt delighted that someone back home remembered her.

"I just can't do it anymore" . . . "I've got to get out of nursing" . . . "I hate it" . . . these are cries for help. Your physical and emotional health is just as important as your patients'. Ask for help when you need it.

SET REALISTIC GOALS

Lily Tomlin once said: "If I had known what it would cost me to have it all, I would have settled for less" (James, 1993, p. 69). Let go of the myth that anyone has it all. Excellence? Yes. Perfection? No. There's a difference. A nursing instructor asks: "Why is it we teach our students to allow their patients to progress at their own speed, but then we deny the students that privilege?" Develop a personal style that is comfortable for you and you alone.

ACCEPT WHAT YOU HAVE NO POWER TO CHANGE

In their delightful book, *Having Our Say: The Delany Sisters' First 100 Years* (Delany & Delany, 1993, p. 115), wise Bessie said: "When I was young nothing could hold me back. It took me a hundred years to figure out I *can't* change the world. I can only change Bessie. And, honey, that ain't easy either."

While it's true there are some aspects of our jobs that we can't change, don't let that wear you down. Deep inside every nurse is the desire to make a special contribution. No one is just another nurse. How much of a difference can one nurse actually make, you may wonder? A significant one. Every kindness you extend, every junior nurse you precept, pays rich dividends as the years roll by. It's an investment that can't be measured in dollars.

When things are tense, though, it's often a sign that a change is needed. "Instead of succumbing to complaining—nursing's favorite indoor sport," says a nursing supervisor, "explore if a change might well begin with you." That's far better than resigning yourself to the idea that you're doing the best you can.

IF YOU'RE IN A RUT, GET OUT OF IT

"The people who seem the most unhappy are the ones whose time is taken up by too much that is repetitive, routine, and ultimately uncreative," says Alexandra Stoddard (1994, p. 179). Nurses? Yes. So much of what we do is determined by rules, regulations, routines, and tradition.

"All some nurses want to do is sit at home and have the hospital mail them a paycheck," argues one nurse. But is this really the case, or could it indicate burnout? When your work focuses primarily on problems or negatives, or when you rarely receive feedback that you are doing a good job, you are a prime candidate for burnout. And employee burnout is a major threat to customer satisfaction (Scott, 1991).

Boredom is another snuffer of workplace satisfaction. That's why it's vital to have a full life outside of nursing. If you're bored with life in general, you'll likely be bored with nursing and too narrowly focused. Pursue outside interests. Expand your knowledge base beyond the confines of the world of nursing. There is much to be learned from others. Instead of "awfulizing" about the way things could or should be, read and study outside your chosen profession. It really changes your perspective.

"If your daily life seems poor," wrote the poet Rilke (1934, pp. 19-20), "do not blame it; blame yourself, tell yourself that you are not poet enough to call forth its riches; for to the creator there is no poverty and no poor indifferent place."

LOOK FOR HIDDEN STRENGTHS IN YOUR COWORKERS

Prisoners of war who are isolated in solitary confinement recognize early on the tremendous strength in unity. "You'd be surprised at the smart stuff that's said when we tune into each other," says a day care nurse. Take time to figure out what's right with nursing. We often sell ourselves short.

Perhaps that graduate nurse technician came to nursing with a teaching degree. Or that nursing assistant on the evening shift, doesn't he head up the annual Heart Fund drive? Take a look around your department. Do some of your staff work in leadership roles in the community, church, sports? All nursing personnel are gifted in some way. It may be they all haven't opened up their gifts yet.

And when a credible coworker has done an incredible job, nominate them for "Employee of the Year" or another appropriate honor in your agency. Show your coworkers you care personally about them. This doesn't necessarily mean showering them with expensive gifts. One nurse who recently moved to Lexington, Kentucky, was amazed at a gentle gesture of the staff on her unit. "They brew gourmet coffee here for no reason at all," she said. "What a treat!" The unity of a team spirit makes a palpable difference. In healthcare, the whole really is greater than the sum of its parts.

When workers don't bolster each other's strengths, it's a barrier to productivity, and leads to a rise in errors and customer dissatisfaction as well. Be a mentor—not a tormentor—to that new nurse who transferred from another doctor's office across town. So what if she does things a little differently? You don't need to walk on water and change healthcare in a Third World country to be an excellent nurse. Treat your colleagues like they're some of your most important customers. They are.

REASSESS YOUR GOALS FREQUENTLY

The time of your annual performance appraisal is a good time to reevaluate your competency and progress, and to examine both your short- and long-term goals. Still, the once a year proficiency is insufficient feedback for any nurse. The most important feedback is what you tell yourself and receive from your customers and coworkers.

BELIEVE IN YOURSELF

We nurses have been well schooled in doubting our abilities. Maybe you fall into the doubting trap yourself. As one critical care nurse said, "If they ever give an Olympic gold medal for self-doubt, a nurse will win it hands down." If we don't believe in ourselves, how can we expect others to?

If you're having difficulty in the doubt department, remind yourself of your positive attributes every day as you drive home from work. Act as if you feel positive about yourself—but not in an artificial way, of course. Feeling often follows action.

DARE TO BE DIFFERENT

Being different takes courage. Many nurses have never developed a taste for risk-taking. "I have too many bills to pay to take chances," says an evening shift nurse. "Especially in this day and time when they send nurses home without pay for low patient census."

When a cat gets burned skittering across a stove burner, he doesn't just avoid the hot coils in the future. He avoids the stove. That's what's happened to a lot of nurses. Consequently, many have an investment in the way things are.

While being creative may be irritating to some people, and originality scorned, don't be bound to what others think. You don't have to live 50 miles from the flagpole to be an expert. Brainstorm with your peers to get your collective creative juices flowing.

Walt Disney didn't get pumped up about any idea unless all his board members had resisted it. He contended that if people supported an idea initially, there wouldn't be sufficient energy to see it through to completion (Shaughnessy, 1993).

It is always somewhat scary to go against the grain. In nursing what is so often lacking is the freedom to fail. We don't want to get labeled as a "troublemaker" or someone whose ideas are contaminated.

Brown and coauthors, while they are not nurses, (1993), who aren't nurses, suggest a "threat-free" work environment where employees are actually encouraged to take risks. This establishes a climate of creativity because mistakes—the natural consequences to creative thinking—are not punished. Interestingly, when people are given the freedom to fail, they actually make fewer errors than in a more restrictive environment. Unfortunately, nursing so rarely empowers people who are different.

MAKE A MEMORY

Remember the ingredients of a successful family? They spent leisure time together. They celebrated the small stuff of everyday life. Establish some traditions with your coworkers—an annual covered-dish holiday meal, perhaps. "It's a way of treating each other like we're special—not like some disposable piece of equipment," says one nurse. Simple respect and consideration are great memory makers.

Think back to your favorite childhood memories . . . a birthday party with all your school chums. Someone was responsible for making that memory happen. Likewise, memories with our colleagues are usually the result of a conscious effort. One group of nurses has a tradition that when anyone goes out of town to a continuing education offering, they bring back a pretty cup and saucer. Every few months, they celebrate afternoon tea. The clinking china cups—all as different as the nurses who chose them—make a positive statement about nursing's beautiful diversity.

KNOW WHEN TO SAY "NO"

You're the CEO of your own life. Learn how to say "No," often the longest word in the English language. Learn, also, to listen to your limitations. A need isn't necessarily a call. If there's not enough of you left to fix dinner for your in-laws after doubling back to day shift, just say "No" . . . and without the guilt. That's not being selfish; it's just taking care of yourself.

When day-to-day life is out of balance, people often try to achieve that balance by doing less or demanding more. Simplify when you feel tugged at every turn. Hire someone to clean your house so you can have time to enjoy the holidays.

Saying "No" at the right times means saying "Yes" to those things that really count. Succeeding in nursing (or anything else) is no success at all if you foolishly push the important things to the side. Don't fall prey to the myth that everyone else is doing it all. "We're always in school," says a nurse who just completed her MSN. "Why are we so driven? We work as much as we can without dropping over, then get up the next day and start right in again. Pretty soon, we're no good to anyone except as a tragic illustration."

LIVE IN THE MOMENT

When you yearn for the day when the ideal job and circumstances have come your way, you sacrifice your own personal development and may even make bad choices. Life is a series of moments. Invest in those ordinary moments. Be the best you can be. Every day is a lifetime in miniature. Don't be like the bumper sticker that reads: "Having a wonderful time. Wish I were here."

What would be your ideal day or evening off? Give yourself the present of that soul-soothing luxury. Write it on your calendar as if it were a date with a close friend. It is. If you can't afford to go away, plan a vacation right at home. Find an overnight sitter. Take the phone off the hook. Stock your refrigerator with comfort foods and break out your best dishes and silver. Snuggle up with that book you've been wanting to read. Let the nurturing begin ... lifestyles of the not so rich and famous.

Take time for leisure. Recreation is re-creation. Play as hard as you work. It isn't being self-indulgent or a waste of time. We should be human beings, not human doings.

DON'T JUDGE YOUR COWORKERS
BY UNREALISTIC STANDARDS

A nurse tells the story about the time she borrowed her husband's power screwdriver to mount a shelf on her kitchen wall. "It was crooked," she admits with a chuckle. "When my husband saw it, he commented, 'If I had done that job, you would have made me do it over.' Funny thing is, I was satisfied with it. It's amazing how our standards go down when we do the work ourselves." Good advice in the nursing arena, too.

"We sabotage each other on my unit. It's just pick, pick, pick," says a night shift charge nurse. "It's one of our profession's fatal flaws." Sure, it cuts deep when a nurse we've tried to help back-stabs us. But try not to let it penetrate you at an emotional level. Nursing, at its best, is difficult. Turn a freeing corner and forgive. Every time we invalidate each other, we weaken the profession. Give a trying coworker the gift of a clean slate. And remember, in the changing world of healthcare, we're all in this together. Try to avoid personalizing critical comments which may reflect frustration or a systems problem, not your personal deficit.

Jakob Boehme (1994, p. 70) observed: "The flowers of the earth do not grudge at one another, though one be more beautiful and fuller of virtue than another; but they stand kindly one by another, and enjoy another's virtue." Oh, for nursing to learn that lesson from nature . . . living each day as if it were our last day, loving those around us because we've learned first to love ourselves.

References

Boehme, J. (1994, March). The language of flowers. *Victoria*, 70.

Brodeur, D. (1995). Work ethics and CQI. *Hospital and Health Services Administration* (special CQI issue), *40*(1), 111-123.

Brown, S. W., Nelson, A. M., Bronkesh, S. J., & Wood, S. D. (1993). *Patient satisfaction pays: Quality service for practice success.* Gaithersburg, MD: Aspen Publishers, Inc.

Buhler, R. (1991). *New choices new boundaries.* Nashville: Thomas Nelson Publishers.

Cook, M. (1992). *Freeing your creativity: A writer's guide.* Cincinnati, OH: Writer's Digest Books.

Crabb, L. (1990). Foreword. In R. Crabb, *The personal touch: Encouraging others through hospitality.* Colorado Springs: Nav Press.

Delany, S., & Delany, A. E. (1993). *Having our say: The Delany sisters' first 100 years.* New York: Kodansha International.

Family Circle Family Index. (1993, Nov. 23). Secrets of successful families. *Family Circle,* 81.

Geisel, T. S., & Geisel, A. S. (1971). *The lorax.* New York: Random House.

Heymann, T. (1991). *In an average lifetime.* New York: Fawcett Columbine.

James, J. (1993). *Visions from the heart.* New York: Newmarket Press.

McFarland, J. R. (1993). *Now that I have cancer I am whole.* Kansas City: Andrews and McMeel.

Melum, M. M, & Sinioris, M. (1989, Feb. 5). The next generation of health care quality. *Hospitals,* 80.

Moran, R. A. (1993). *Never confuse a memo with reality (and other business lessons too simple not to know)*. New York: Harper Collins Publishers.

Nachmanovitch, S. (1990). *Free play*. New York: G.P. Putnam's Sons.

Pearson, P. (1991). *You deserve the best*. Dallas: Connemara Press.

Rilke, R. M. (1934). *Letters to a young poet*. New York: W.W. Norton and Company.

Rosenbluth, H. F., & Peters, D. M. (1992). *The customer comes second and other secrets of exceptional service*. New York: Quill (William Morrow & Co.).

Scott, D. (1991). *Customer satisfaction: The other half of your job*. Menlo Park, CA: Crisp Publications, Inc.

Shaughnessy, S. (1993). *Walking on alligators: A book of meditations for writers*. New York: Harper Collins Publishers.

Stoddard, A. (1994). *Making choices: The joy of a courageous life*. New York: William Morrow & Co., Inc.

Summers, C. (1994). Self-care: The greatest challenge for nurses. *Revolution: The Journal of Nurse Empowerment, 4*(3), 93-96.

APPENDIX

Sample Patient Satisfaction Survey

HOW ARE WE DOING?

(Sample Patient Satisfaction Questionnaire)

(This example, which provides a variety of sample questions that integrate the key principles highlighted in this book, can be adapted to outpatient and community settings including physicians' offices, clinics, same-day surgery centers, HMOs, etc. *Your* satisfaction survey should take into consideration the mission, vision, and values of your institution, as pertinent to those you serve, and not merely the administration of your facility. You will want to tailor this questionnaire to the literacy level of your patient population. You may also wish to use the headings provided only for data analysis.)

INSTRUCTIONS: Please answer these questions about your recent stay at Hometown Hospital. For each question, indicate the number which best describes your level of satisfaction. The number 1 means Excellent, 2 means Very Good, 3 means Good, 4 means Fair, and 5 means Poor.

If a question does not apply, mark N/A (non-applicable).

Your answers are confidential and will be used to improve our care and services in the future. Please share any comments, either good or bad, in the spaces provided. If you have any questions, please call Ima Friend, the patient representative, at (555) 555-5555.

When you have finished the questionnaire, mail it to the Director of Patient Relations in the self-addressed, stamped envelope.

Thank you for your help.

	Excellent	Very Good	Good	Fair	Poor	N/A
Ease of Admissions Procedure:						
1. The time it took from when you arrived at the hospital until you were taken to your room.	1	2	3	4	5	☐

Comments: _____

_____

	Excellent	Very Good	Good	Fair	Poor	N/A
Your Doctor						
2. Trust in the skill and ability of your doctor.	1	2	3	4	5	☐
3. The number of times your doctor came to see you.	1	2	3	4	5	☐

Comments: _____

_____

	Excellent	Very Good	Good	Fair	Poor	N/A
Your Nurses						
4. Trust in the skill and ability of your nurses.	1	2	3	4	5	☐
5. The number of times a nurse checked on you to see how you were doing.	1	2	3	4	5	☐
6. Your feelings/opinions were considered in planning your care.	1	2	3	4	5	☐
7. Your call light was answered quickly.	1	2	3	4	5	☐
8. Pain medication was given on time and helped your pain.	1	2	3	4	5	☐
9. Help with eating, bathing, dressing, getting into a chair, and going to the bathroom was given quickly when you asked.	1	2	3	4	5	☐

Comments: _____

_____

	Excellent	Very Good	Good	Fair	Poor	N/A
Other Hospital Staff						
10. Trust in the skill and ability of other hospital workers who helped take care of you (such as laboratory, x-ray, food service, respiratory care, social services, pharmacy, physical therapy, transport, etc.).	1	2	3	4	5	☐

	Excellent	Very Good	Good	Fair	Poor	N/A
11. Hospital staff worked together well.	1	2	3	4	5	☐
12. All hospital workers made sure your privacy was respected.	1	2	3	4	5	☐
13. Your minister, priest, rabbi, or the hospital chaplain was able to visit as you needed.	1	2	3	4	5	☐

Comments: _____

_____

Your Daily Care

14. Hospital workers were polite, helpful, respectful, and were there when you needed them.	1	2	3	4	5	☐
15. Your special needs and desires were taken care of.	1	2	3	4	5	☐
16. Food was of good quality and was served at the right temperature.	1	2	3	4	5	☐
17. You were treated in a kind, caring, and friendly way.	1	2	3	4	5	☐

Comments: _____

_____

The Hospital Environment

18. Your room was clean, had good lighting, wasn't too hot or too cold, and was quiet.	1	2	3	4	5	☐
19. The TV, telephone, lights, bed controls, and call button worked and were easy to reach.	1	2	3	4	5	☐

	Excellent	Very Good	Good	Fair	Poor	N/A
20. Signs and directions were easy to follow.	1	2	3	4	5	☐
21. You found a parking space and it wasn't too far away.	1	2	3	4	5	☐

Comments: _____

_____

Your Family

	Excellent	Very Good	Good	Fair	Poor	N/A
22. Your family and visitors were treated in a kind, caring, and friendly way.	1	2	3	4	5	☐
23. Your family had a nice waiting area.	1	2	3	4	5	☐
24. Visiting times were good for your family.	1	2	3	4	5	☐
25. The people you wanted to know about your stay were kept up-to-date while you were in the hospital.	1	2	3	4	5	☐

Comments: _____

_____

Patient Education

	Excellent	Very Good	Good	Fair	Poor	N/A
26. Tests, treatments, diet, use of equipment, and medications were explained in a way you could understand.	1	2	3	4	5	☐
27. Results of tests, treatments, medications, and procedures were explained in a way you could understand.	1	2	3	4	5	☐

Comments: _____

_____

	Excellent	Very Good	Good	Fair	Poor	N/A

Preparation for Discharge

28. Discharge instructions were clear and complete.

    1   2   3   4   5   ☐

29. Information was given about possible problems to watch for after you went home.

    1   2   3   4   5   ☐

30. You could understand the instructions the hospital gave you when you were discharged.

    1   2   3   4   5   ☐

31. Referrals to community services and/or your private doctor were made if needed.

    1   2   3   4   5   ☐

Comments: _____

_____

Your Bill

32. Your hospital bill was received right away, was correct, and was easy to understand.

    1   2   3   4   5   ☐

Comments: _____

_____

Overall Satisfaction

33. How happy you were with your stay at Hometown Hospital.

    1   2   3   4   5   ☐

Comments: _____

_____

GENERAL INFORMATION
(Please fill in the blanks)

34. Will you return to Hometown Hospital again?   ☐ YES   ☐ NO

35. Will you recommend Hometown Hospital to others?   ☐ YES   ☐ NO

36. If you could change one thing about your stay, what would it be?
    Describe: _____
    _____

37. Did anything happen, good or bad, that you had not expected?
    Describe: _____
    _____

38. How have you gotten better as a result of your stay at Hometown Hospital?
    Describe: _____
    _____

39. At any time did you feel your condition was discussed with someone you
    did not want to have that information?
    If yes, explain: _____
    _____

40. Have you been a patient at this hospital before? _____
    If yes, how many times?_____

41. Why were you admitted to the hospital?_____
    _____

42. How long were you in the hospital this time?_____

43. What is your age?_____

44. How far do you live from the hospital?_____

45. Are you male or female? _____

46. Would you be willing to talk about your stay at Hometown Hospital with a
    group of other patients?   ☐ YES   ☐ NO

47. Your name (not required)_____

INDEX